AIDS & *the Impact of* Cognitive Impairment

A Treatment Guide for Mental Health Providers

Penelope Zeifert, PhD
Mark Leary, MD
Alicia A. Boccellari, PhD

UCSF AIDS Health Project Monograph Series Number One
Published by the AIDS Health Project, University of California San Francisco

INFORMATION. UCSF AIDS Health Project, Box 0884, San Francisco, CA 94143-0884.

First Printing, June 1995. Printed in the United States of America

LIBRARY OF CONGRESS CATALOGING-IN-PUBLICATION DATA

Zeifert, Penelope. 1948-

AIDS and the impact of cognitive impairment : a treatment guide for mental health providers / Penelope Zeifert, Mark Leary, and Alicia A. Boccellari.

p. cm. – (UCSF AHP monograph ; no. 1)

Includes bibliographical references and index.

ISBN 1-879168-01-4 (trade pbk.)

1. Brain–Infections–Complications. 2. AIDS dementia complex. 3. AIDS (Disease)–Patients–Mental health. 4. Cognition disorders.

I. Leary, Mark, 1955- . II. Boccellari, Alicia A., 1955- . III. Title. IV. Series.

[DNLM: 1. Cognition Disorders–therapy. 2. Cognition Disorders–etiology. 3. Acquired Immunodeficiency Syndrome–complications. WM 204 Z46a 1995]

RC359.5.Z45 1995

616.8–dc20

DNLM/DLC

for Library of Congress 95-35959

CIP

UCSF AIDS HEALTH PROJECT. James W. Dilley, MD, Executive Director.

Robert Marks, Director of Publications, Editor. Michal Longfelder, Outreach and Marketing. Saul Rosenfield, Cover, Book design. Sayre Van Young, Indexing. Kelly Van Noord, Production. Kathy Barr, Benjamin Steele, Jennifer Cohen, Proofreading. Sandra Kriletich, Distribution. Stephen Follansbee, MD, George Harrison, MD, Robin Ortiz, James Dotson, MD, Manuscript review. John Tighe, Editorial assistance. Jennifer Cohen, Administrative support. Julie Balovich, Shirley Gibson, Mark Kuhnle, Research and production support.

DONATIONS AND GRANTS. Typefaces donated by Adobe Systems, Mountain View, California. Cover illustration adapted by permission, Webster's Third New International Dictionary © 1986 Merriam-Webster, Inc. We thank these companies for their generosity.

Funding for this book from the California Department of Mental Health: Pete Wilson, Governor; Russell Gould, Secretary, Health and Welfare Agency; D. William Mayer, MD, Director of Mental Health, California Department of Mental Health.

DISCLAIMER. Please note: the names used in the case scenarios in this book are fictitious.

Contents

Contributors

PENELOPE ZEIFERT, PhD is an Assistant Clinical Professor of Psychiatry at the University of California San Francisco (UCSF) and a clinical neuropsychologist at Stanford University, Stanford University Hospital, and Laguna Honda Hospital in San Francisco.

MARK LEARY, MD is Deputy Chief of Psychiatry at San Francisco General Hospital (SFGH) and an Assistant Clinical Professor of Psychiatry at UCSF. He is Co-Chair of the SFGH Psychiatry HIV Task Force and a member of the statewide AIDS Advisory Panel to Health Net (a health maintenance organization).

ALICIA A. BOCCELLARI, PHD is Director of the Neuropsychology Service and the Division of Psychosocial Medicine at SFGH and an Associate Clinical Professor of Psychology at UCSF. Dr. Boccellari has worked with HIV disease since 1985, as a clinician and researcher and has lectured and published widely on the topic.

UCSF AIDS Health Project Monograph Series

THE UCSF AIDS HEALTH PROJECT, affiliated with the Langley Porter Psychiatric Institute of the University of California San Francisco's world-renowned medical school, has been a leader in developing clinical services and professional education to meet the mental health needs of people affected by HIV disease. Since 1984, AHP has been nationally recognized for pioneering programs in a variety of areas including HIV-related counseling and support, antibody testing and counseling, and HIV-related substance abuse services.

AHP publishes *FOCUS: A Guide to AIDS Research and Counseling,* one of the longest-running HIV-related newsletters in the country, and other books and newsletters on HIV-related counseling. The UCSF AIDS Health Project Monograph Series, underwritten by the California Department of Mental Health, offers clear, concise, and practical information on HIV-related topics of particular concern to mental health providers.

Acknowledgments

Putting a monograph like this together requires the efforts of many people. The authors wish to acknowledge especially the following people, but they and the editors extend their appreciation to UCSF AIDS Health Project staff and volunteers who contributed to the process. (See the copyright page for a list of these individuals.)

I wish to thank my co-authors: Alicia Boccellari for her mentorship and her conceptualization of the cognitive impairment management model, and Mark Leary, without whose writing partnership this monograph would not have been possible. Throughout numerous revisions, he produced quality work and maintained a sense of humor and perspective. Peter Goldblum, PhD, MPH provided valuable information on his psychotherapeutic approach. Ron Patten, LCSW contributed his impressive knowledge of social service systems in devising a model for locating community resources. James Dilley, MD and Gary Grossman, PhD provided clinical expertise on HIV-related issues. Stephen Follansbee, MD, George Harrison, MD, and Robin Ortiz reviewed the manuscript and offered insightful feedback. Rob Marks, our editor, was remarkably patient and persevering. Sue von Bayer, PhD taught me to use a Macintosh computer and, at deadline, gave me use of her computer and house for two long days. Alice Tompkins generously lent me her laptop so I could do revisions wherever I happened to be. Linda Lagemann, PhD provided a valuable read-through and helped me organize and rewrite for clarity and emphasis. Finally, my family took in stride my absences and my preoccupation and offered me loving respite from the work.

– Penelope Zeifert, PhD

I want to acknowledge our editor Rob Marks for his patience, care, and diligence in focusing our efforts, and Stephen Follansbee, MD and George Harrison, MD for their thoughtful comments in reviewing the manuscript. James Dilley, MD has provided inspiration, direction, and wise suggestions from the very beginning of the process of writing this book. The monograph would not have been possible without the contribution of patients with HIV infection in the Psychiatry Department of San Francisco General Hospital, with whom I have been privileged to work over the past six years. They have taught me much of what I know about the psychiatric and cognitive aspects of HIV infection. As always, it has been a distinct pleasure to work with Penelope Zeifert and Alicia Boccellari. I look forward to continuing to learn from them in the future. Finally, I want to thank my wife, Jeanne Burns Leary, MD, whose support and enthusiasm has sustained me throughout the project.

– Mark Leary, MD

I wish to thank Michael Shore, PhD for his ongoing support and consultation. His advice has been central in helping me conceptualize and understand HIV-associated dementia and develop treatment strategies to respond to it. I also wish to thank Penelope Zeifert and Mark Leary for their commitment to seeing this project through; it could not have been accomplished without their dedication. Finally, I wish to thank the patients, family members, and caregivers who have so willingly shared their experiences with me. I have learned so much from them and feel so privileged to have been allowed into their lives.

– Alicia A. Boccellari, PhD

Introduction

AIDS threatens the mind as well as the body. Through a variety of mechanisms, HIV disease can bring about changes in thought, emotion, and behavior, leading to symptoms of "cognitive impairment," the loss of the ability to process, learn, and remember information. The result is a confusing array of changes in behavior and cognition that becomes apparent in the course of providing psychotherapy to HIV-infected clients and that inspires fear and helplessness in both clients and providers.

Mental health training does not prepare providers for the demanding task of assessing cognitive impairment, determining psychotherapeutic approaches and goals in the face of both mild and significant cognitive impairment, and clarifying the role of friends, family members, and partners in treatment. This monograph seeks to provide mental health and medical practitioners with a road map of the disorders that cause impairment and a pathway to follow toward accurate diagnosis and appropriate treatment. It also outlines the necessary information to educate clients and the ways to respond to the needs of the families and friends of clients with cognitive impairment.

As a practical clinical guide, the monograph describes the process through which provider and client might go to discover and respond to impairment. The first chapter describes the range of conditions that can cause impairment, including: direct HIV infection of the brain, HIV-related opportunistic conditions that affect neural function, organic mood disorders* like depression and mania, and HIV-related treatments themselves. This chapter includes a description of incidence, signs and symptoms, pathophysiology, and diagnostic work-up. The second chapter offers a primer on the diagnostic tools and process useful to clarify the causes of cognitive impairment.

The third chapter focuses on the treatment and management of cognitive impairment symptoms, including information on psychotherapy, coordination of treatment with psychiatry, psychopharmacology, and for the more significantly cognitively impaired, environmental and behavioral interventions. Finally, because the effects of cognitive impairment extend beyond clients themselves, the fourth chapter briefly covers two important issues for both providers and caregivers: stress and countertransference.†

As always, knowledge sheds light. For both providers and clients, understanding the scope of impairment, the intractable limitations it may pose, and the many adaptations that may be reached can offer comfort and maintain quality of life and human dignity.

---

* The American Psychiatric Association's Diagnostic and Statistical Manual of Mental Disorders, Fourth Edition (DSM-IV) no longer uses the term "Organic Affective Disorder" to refer to a mood disorder that is seen as a "result of the direct physiological consequence of a general medical condition." Instead, the DSM-IV uses designations such as "Dementia Due to HIV Disease, with Depressed Mood." Despite the change, the monograph continues to observe common usage: "organic affective disorder" or "organic mood disorder."

† Throughout the text of the monograph, the term "caregiver" refers to partners, family members, and friends of people with HIV disease – individuals who provide care as non-professionals.

1

Causes of Cognitive Impairment

HIV-related cognitive changes are caused by a variety of conditions. The most common cause is direct infection of the brain by HIV, which may result in HIV-associated dementia. Other causes include opportunistic conditions such as toxoplasmosis and lymphoma; organic affective disorders such as mania and depression; and conditions that lead to transient impairment such as delirium and substance abuse.

Some aspects of cognitive impairment are treatable if addressed quickly; others are untreatable and rapidly progressive. When cognitive impairment occurs among people with HIV disease, more than one disorder may be present, a situation that complicates assessment and treatment.

Direct Infection of the Brain by HIV

Summary

- Most HIV-related cognitive impairment is caused by direct infection of the brain. Two conditions result from infection: "HIV-associated minor cognitive/motor disorder," at the mild end of the impairment continuum, and "HIV-associated dementia," at the severe end. HIV-associated dementia is an AIDS-defining condition.
- Cognitive impairment occurs in 55 percent to 65 percent of people with AIDS. The most severe aspects of HIV-related cognitive impairment occur in the later stages of HIV infection as the immune system becomes more suppressed. Other co-factors include: low weight, constitutional symptoms, and anemia (low hemoglobin values).
- HIV infects the brain by crossing the blood-brain barrier in "macrophages," infection-fighting blood cells. It causes impairment by damaging the "myelin," the "white matter" of the brain, a fatty substance that insulates the branches of neurons and facilitates electrochemical conduction of nerve impulses.
- Diagnosis of HIV-associated dementia requires fulfilling three criteria: a positive HIV antibody test confirming HIV infection; confirmation of disabling cognitive, motor, or behavioral symptoms that interfere with occupational or social functioning; and the exclusion of other potential causes of cognitive impairment, for example, toxoplasmosis, vitamin B_{12} deficiency, or substance abuse.
- It is the degree of impairment in activities of daily living and the resulting impact on independence that distinguishes HIV-associated dementia from HIV-associated minor cognitive/motor disorder. Among the functions affected by impairment are: concentration, memory, thinking, speech, emotional expression, social behavior, the ability to perform complex tasks, the ability to focus on specific stimuli, coordination and balance, and muscle strength.

HIV-associated dementia is the most prevalent of the HIV-related brain disorders and the condition that mental health providers find the most challenging. It is difficult to determine the presence and degree of cognitive impairment in people with dementia, and psychotherapy in this context is unfamiliar to many practitioners. In contrast to other brain disorders, HIV-associated dementia is caused by direct infection of the brain by HIV itself. It presents with disturbances in cognition, motor function, and behavior. In advanced stages, it profoundly affects an individual's ability to care for him or herself and to participate fully in treatment decisions.[1]

Since its identification in 1983, HIV-associated dementia has been known as "AIDS encephalopathy," "subacute encephalitis," "AIDS encephalitis,"[2] "AIDS dementia complex (ADC)"[3,4] and most recently, "HIV-associated dementia complex" (HAD).[5] The name changes have in part been attempts to describe the phenomenon more clearly. For example, subacute encephalitis reflected the belief that cognitive impairment was caused by acute inflammation of the brain that persisted for an extended period of time. As it became clearer that these symptoms were not caused by inflammation alone, researchers coined "AIDS Dementia Complex" to describe a constellation of symptoms affecting three areas – cognition, motor function, and behavior – that developed late in the course of HIV infection. In 1987, the Centers for Disease Control and Prevention (CDC) added AIDS dementia complex to its list of AIDS-defining disorders, thus acknowledging the importance of the syndrome and confirming its relationship to HIV disease.

Over the past decade, these terms have been used interchangeably to indicate a generally accepted clinical picture of dementia.[6] In 1991, the American Academy of Neurology developed nomenclature and operational definitions to detail criteria for diagnosing HIV-associated dementia. These criteria emphasize the range of cognitive and motor impairment embodied by dementia: "HIV-associated dementia" describes the severe end of the spectrum; and "HIV-associated minor cognitive/motor disorder" describes mild impairment that does not meet the threshold for dementia.[5]

Diagnosis of HIV-associated dementia requires fulfilling three criteria: a positive HIV antibody test confirming HIV infection; disabling cognitive, motor, or behavioral symptoms that interfere with occupational or social functioning; and the exclusion of other potential causes of cognitive impairment, for example, toxoplasmosis, lymphoma of the central nervous system (CNS), vitamin B_{12} deficiency, or substance abuse. Diagnostic evaluation of cognitive impairment itself may entail: laboratory and radiological procedures; neurological examination; neuropsychiatric evaluation, including mental status exam; and neuropsychological testing.

Dementia and The Trojan Horse

The mechanism by which HIV disrupts the functioning of the brain remains unknown. However, neuroscientists have several theories of HIV brain infection and its subsequent damage based on autopsies of HIV-infected brain tissue. To understand these theories, it is important to appreciate the physiology of the brain.

Because of the brain's overriding physiologic importance, it has evolved special defensive systems to protect it from invasion by bacteria, viruses, and other infectious agents. The most important of these systems is the "blood-brain barrier," a tight network of cells that limits entry into the brain only to blood cells it recognizes as "self." HIV appears to circumvent the blood-brain barrier by utilizing an ingenious "Trojan Horse" ploy.[7] As it circulates in the blood, the virus is engulfed by macrophages, the body's normal infection-fighting blood cells. Since the blood-brain barrier cannot distinguish HIV-infected macrophages, it recognizes them as "self" and allows them to enter the brain with HIV concealed inside.

Once in the brain, HIV is able to replicate within the macrophages and other similar immunologic cells called multinucleated giant cells. In individuals with HIV-associated dementia or lesser cognitive impairment, HIV presumably breaks out of its hiding places in the macrophages and multinucleated giant cells. It appears that HIV does not primarily infect the main cell elements of the brain – neurons and oligodendrocytes – to a significant degree. While autopsy studies of HIV dementia show some loss of brain cells, including neurons, this loss is insufficient to explain the severity of clinical symptoms observed in living clients. What appears more important is the commonly observed loss of myelin tissue, also called "white matter." Myelin is a fatty substance that insulates the branches of neurons, facilitating the electrochemical conduction of brain impulses and the quickness with which a person thinks. In this way, HIV appears to disrupt brain functioning and leads to symptoms of cognitive and motor impairment.

Brain scans – magnetic resonance imaging (MRI) and computerized tomography (CT) – of many, but not all, people with HIV dementia or minor cognitive impairment show the loss of brain tissue. This loss of tissue, commonly called atrophy, is most prominent in the areas surrounding the brain's ventricles, spaces normally filled with fluid; but it may also be seen in the cortex, the outer surfaces of the brain, especially in advanced disease. In addition, brain scans typically reveal abnormalities of the myelin, particularly in the centrally-located area beneath the cortex (called the "subcortex"), particularly the basal ganglia (the centers controlling motor function) and the thalamus (an area that integrates the different functions required to perform complex tasks).

Chemical Sabotage of Nerve Cells

Studies have implicated several chemical substances as instruments of HIV-related nerve cell degeneration. At least two protein components of HIV damage the outer membranes covering nerve cells. The two proteins, gp120 ("glycoprotein 120," a molecule that makes up a portion of the outer coat of the virus) and tat (short for "transactivator," a protein within the virus) change the permeability of nerve cell membranes. This may change the chemical balance inside nerve cells, disrupting their normal function and leading to cell damage or death. In one study, high levels of gp120 were found to be associated with abnormally elevated levels of calcium within nerve cells. This latter finding has prompted research into nimodipine, a drug that blocks the entry of calcium into cells, as a treatment for HIV-associated dementia.[8]

Other studies suggest that cytokines, chemicals produced by macrophages and glial brain cells in response to HIV infection, may themselves damage nerve cells. These naturally occurring substances – called interleukin-1, interleukin-6, neopterin, and tumor necrosis factor alpha – are part of the body's normal immune response to infection and disease. However, HIV brain infection appears to subvert this response: cytokines actually have a toxic effect, presumably interfering with nerve cell conduction, causing clinical symptoms of HIV dementia and cognitive impairment. Other chemicals generated by the immune system in response to HIV brain infection, including $beta_2$ microglobulin and quinolinic acid, have been associated with the disruption of brain cell functioning. For example, it appears that quinolinic acid interacts with a specialized chemical receptor in nerve cell membranes to cause dysfunction.

While autopsy studies suggest that HIV is present in the brains of more than 90 percent of people with AIDS at the time of death, a smaller percentage of people with AIDS appear to develop HIV-associated dementia or minor cognitive/motor disorder. Researchers offer several theories for this, including: different strains of HIV have different propensities to disrupt brain functioning; genetic variations make some individuals more susceptible to the effects of HIV brain infection; and pre-existing conditions – for example, prior brain infection, trauma, or drug use – make some people more vulnerable.

Epidemiology and Natural History

The epidemiology and natural history of HIV-associated cognitive impairment have not yet been clearly defined. It is generally accepted that dementia occurs in conjunction with immunosuppression. Late in the course of HIV infection, a significant number of individuals have some degree of cognitive impairment, although it may not meet the criteria for HIV-associated dementia.[9] A recent review of the literature estimates that the median prevalence of cognitive impairment among people with AIDS is 55 percent to 65 percent.[7,10]

There is controversy about the extent to which cognitive impairment is present in people who are HIV-infected but not immune suppressed.[11] Some researchers have found subtle cognitive impairment among some asymptomatic HIV-infected people. Other researchers have found no differences in cognition between uninfected and asymptomatic people. Even those who support the view that cognitive impairment may occur early in the course of HIV infection acknowledge that the degree of impairment is subtle and not discernible in activities of daily living.[12] This controversy may in part be due to a lack of clarity regarding the term "asymptomatic." There has been variation in the characteristics defining asymptomatic subjects, and this lack of standardization may have compromised the consistency of results across studies.

The progression of HIV-related cognitive impairment is also unclear. Originally the course was considered to be an invariable decline in function over time.[4] "Dementia" was used to describe any degree of HIV-related cognitive symptomatology; terms clarifying the degree of impairment – mild and severe deficits, early and late stage – were used intermittently. Currently, however, progression is not considered orderly or predictable. HIV-associated minor cognitive/motor disorder and HIV-associated dementia may exist not just as poles on the continuum of HIV-related cognitive impairment, but also as separate entities,[5] and people with HIV-associated minor cognitive/motor disorder may remain functional throughout the course of illness.

The historical overinclusiveness and variability in diagnosis of dementia have led to a wide discrepancy in estimates of the prevalence of HIV-related cognitive impairment.[11] A review of neuropsychiatric studies estimates a prevalence of all HIV-related cognitive impairment at 33 percent to 87 percent among patients with symptomatic HIV disease, and a prevalence of HIV-associated dementia at 8 percent to 16 percent among people with AIDS.[13] A large longitudinal study found that 15 percent of patients with AIDS in the United States developed HIV-associated dementia.[14] The first extensive neuropsychiatric study in developing countries found a prevalence rate of HIV-associated dementia of 5.4 percent to 6.9 percent among symptomatic patients.[15] Researchers conjecture that this is lower than the rate in industrialized countries because of a lack of medical intervention that may lead to an earlier death before progression to dementia.

A diagnosis of AIDS due either to an AIDS-defining illness or a T-helper cell count below 200 is generally considered a precondition to HIV-associated dementia. While absolute T-helper cell level correlates poorly with HIV-related cognitive impairment, the rate of T-helper cell decline is associated with poorer neuropsychological performance.[16] $Beta_2$ microglobulin, neopterin, and quinolinic acid levels may also be a better predictor of impaired neuropsychological functioning than absolute T-helper cell counts.[17,18,19]

Co-factors for rapid development of HIV-associated dementia include anemia, low weight, and other constitutional symptoms. The single best predictor may be lower hemoglobin values.[14] Some studies have found that lower education[15,20] or prior head injury[21] are co-factors for the expression of HIV-related cognitive impairment. This provides some support to the "threshold theory," which proposes that individuals with a lower IQ, or a history of environmental deprivation, poor nutrition, or brain insults have less cognitive reserve or brain resiliency to compensate for brain impairment.[22] These individuals may harbor an underlying structural or neurochemical vulnerability to subsequent brain insults such as HIV-related cognitive impairment.

Clinical Presentation

HIV-associated dementia is characterized by disabling cognitive impairment and is usually accompanied by motor and behavioral dysfunction. In some cases either motor or behavioral abnormalities may be missing, or one may predominate over the other. Regardless of the pattern, the essential feature in HIV-associated dementia is significant functional impairment in work and activities of daily life.

It is the degree of impairment in activities of daily living and the resulting impact on independence that distinguishes HIV-associated dementia from HIV-associated minor cognitive/motor disorder. The latter is characterized by mild cognitive impairment and interference with only the most complex or demanding of daily tasks.

For clinical purposes, it is useful to conceive of HIV-related cognitive impairment as a spectrum moving from mild deficits through severe dementia.[7] However, as stated previously, it is unclear whether the two diagnoses, HIV-associated dementia and HIV-associated minor cognitive/motor disorder, actually exist as two distinct clinical entities or whether they are simply two points along the spectrum of a single disease entity. Regardless, it is important to note that progression through the continuum is not orderly and people may stabilize at different levels of impairment. (See Table 1: Spectrum of HIV-Related Neuropsychiatric Impairment, pages 12-13.)

HIV-associated minor cognitive/motor disorder reflects subtle cognitive impairment that causes only mild interference with work or activities of daily living (ADL). Although individuals with this disorder are able to continue functioning, for the most part, without interruption to normal routine, they are likely to notice and complain about decreased efficiency and difficulty concentrating and remembering. They may also complain of changes in motor function, such as sloppy handwriting. They are especially apt to experience difficulties when faced with novel or demanding circumstances, particularly in the workplace. Stressful situations are more likely than they had been to elicit irritability or emotional distress. Individuals with this level of cognitive impairment may naturally begin to compensate for deficits, for example, by making lists or by decreasing involvement in demanding activities.

When symptoms significantly interfere with work and social functioning, the diagnosis elevates to HIV-associated dementia. This means that a person experiences at least moderate cognitive impairment and additional motor and behavioral abnormalities. At this point, clients have difficulty concentrating on complex information such as medication regimens. They have memory problems, tending to forget information after 20 to 30 minutes; this may not be immediately obvious as this type of memory loss is due to difficulty retrieving information, and thus cues or reminders will help recall. It may also be difficult to remember disparate information discretely; for example, separate conversations may become merged and remembered as one.

At this moderate stage, individuals may remark that they are slower in their thinking, and they may exhibit longer pauses between speech or decreased spontaneous speech. Their emotional expression may be limited and, when combined with slowness, may mimic depression. On the other hand, moderately impaired individuals tend to have preserved verbal skills and may talk at length, particularly about past experiences. Socially they may appear disinhibited; for example, they may make sexually inappropriate statements, and they may neglect grooming and personal hygiene to some degree. They may show a lack of reaction to events that would usually upset them, or a lack of awareness of deficits.

People with moderate dementia have significant difficulty planning and carrying out complex tasks (for example, cooking), so much so that others become alarmed enough to seek help. They also have difficulty paying attention to pertinent stimuli. As a result they may feel overwhelmed and confused in busy environments such as restaurants or grocery stores. They may also report instances of getting "turned around" and lost even in familiar neighborhoods. Finally, they may have gait, balance, and coordination problems, but these are mild and do not preclude ambulation. They may experience slowed motor speed, decreased muscle strength, and tremor.

Later-stage dementia is characterized by a notably sharp decline in functioning. Clients need 24-hour supervision and active assistance from caretakers to engage in the most basic activities of daily living. There is an obvious neglect of grooming and hygiene. Attention and concentration deficits interfere with the ability to read and even limit the ability to follow a conversation. Short-term memory may be severely impaired, impeding the ability to remember conversations over even a short period of time. Clients may become disoriented. Their thinking becomes simplified. Spontaneous speech may diminish to the point of muteness.

Physically, later-stage dementia incorporates generalized weakness, with the legs affected more than the arms. Ataxia (balance

Table 1. Spectrum of HIV-Related Neuropsychiatric Impairment
Cognitive and behavioral characteristics for impairment stages
Adapted from the Neuropsychiatric AIDS Rating Scale [7,23,24]

	ORIENTATION	MEMORY COGNITION
NORMAL	Fully oriented	Normal
EQUIVOCAL	Fully oriented	Reports subjective memory problems, not clearly seen on testing
MILD	Fully oriented but may have brief episodes of "spaciness"	Mild memory problems for recent events; verifiable on testing
MODERATE	Some disorientation	Recent memory notably impaired; difficulty following plot of a story or conversation; may perseverate (persistently repeat)
SEVERE	Frequent disorientation, worse at night	Severe memory loss, speech repetitive and incoherent at times
END STAGE	Confused and disoriented	May be mute and unresponsive; virtually no memory

Motor	Behavior and Affect	Problem Solving	Daily Activities (ADL's)
Normal	Normal	Can solve every-day problems	Fully independent
Fully ambulatory, may have slightly slowed movements	Normal	May have slight delay in response to novel problems	May have slight impairment in financial dealings
May show balance, coordination, and handwriting difficulties	More irritable and emotionally labile or apathetic and withdrawn	Difficulty planning or completing work, especially complicated or novel tasks	Can do simple daily activities; may need prompting for personal hygiene
General weakness; ambulatory but may require a cane	Some impulsivity or agitated behavior; flat affect or extreme withdrawal; disinhibited social behavior	Requires assistance to carry out simple tasks or instructions; may get lost easily	Needs assistance with personal hygiene, shopping, and cooking
May require assistance to ambulate; may be incontinent	May have psychosis or emotional lability; may have fixed vacant stare	May be unable to follow simple instructions or tasks, even with assistance	Cannot live independently; needs assistance with all activities including dressing and toileting
Bedridden	May be non-responsive or easily agitated by minimal stimuli	No problem-solving ability	Nearly vegetative

problems) may require the use of canes or walkers, and eventually lead to wheelchair use or complete immobility. Clients may experience bowel and bladder incontinence.

HIV-associated dementia complex may be complicated by organic mood disorders, either mania or depression. The risk of an episode of these disorders increases with immunosuppression and is greatest in individuals with moderate to severe cognitive impairment.[25,26] (See Organic Affective Disorders, page 21, for descriptions and diagnostic criteria.)

A Note on Agitation

As clients develop HIV-related cognitive impairment, they may become more irritable and emotional in response to environmental demands. With moderate impairment, situations that are mildly stimulating (for example, being in a grocery store) may cause fear, anxiety, and agitation. Usually these feelings recede when people are placed in more familiar or structured situations. However with increasing HIV-associated dementia, clients may develop unease secondary to disorientation and confusion, and they may become agitated with fleeting delusions. Delusions tend to be simple and may concern care givers or medication. A common delusion in people with dementia is that other people are stealing from them.

Agitation presents as anxiety associated with significant motor restlessness, for example, pacing. It can be evident during depression, psychotic states, delirium, and substance-induced psychosis, as well as during dementing conditions.

Merging and Cueing: The Case of Roberta

Roberta, a 38-year-old White woman, was hospitalized with her second episode of *Pneumocystis carinii* pneumonia (PCP) and placed in a skilled nursing facility while she recovered. She had a T-helper cell count of 36. Early in her hospitalization, she was referred to a neuropsychologist – Dr. Janis Hauer – for assessment of depression, having talked continuously about the recent death of her husband.

On interview at her bedside, Roberta presented as verbal and animated, focusing on her life with her husband and her husband's death, at times becoming tearful about the loss. She denied vegetative symptoms although reported feeling depressed at times. She was alert, "oriented times three," that is, she knew the date, who she was, and where she was. She refused neuropsychological testing, however, stating politely but firmly, "I don't want to spend whatever time I have left doing that."

Asked about her adaptation to the hospital where she would remain for another two weeks, Roberta stated initially that there were no problems since she had been moved from a 20-bed ward to her current semi-private room. She explained that the staff on the open ward had been brusque and uncaring, but that the new nursing staff was much better. This perception was notable, because the same doctors and staff served both areas. Roberta then admitted that there was one orderly she disliked, whom she described as "rough" in bathing her. In addition, she stated that this orderly had removed some candy, a gift from a friend. Roberta tearfully expressed concern that the orderly would retaliate against her for reporting this, but stated that she felt she had to do so because other clients on the unit were sicker and more vulnerable than she.

There was no evidence on interview or by staff report that suggested Roberta might be cognitively impaired, although her immune system was significantly suppressed. Dr. Hauer immediately discussed Roberta's complaint with the attending physician, but the client's description of a brusque and uncaring staff was troublesome, not at all fitting with the psychologist's experience of this staff. Roberta's report suggested symptoms of cognitive impairment, specifically of mental slowing, a propensity to become overwhelmed in a stimulating environment, a lack of awareness of cognitive deficits and, thus, the perception of the etiology as external. The world seemed confusing, noisy, and moving too quickly. A logical way of thinking about this situation was for Roberta to perceive people as curtly rushing her.

When Dr. Hauer returned to Roberta's room, the client was welcoming. She said that she remembered Dr. Hauer, but not her name or position. Dr. Hauer noticed what was obviously a candy box on a table, covered by some papers. In response to a comment about the candy, Roberta became animated, stating it had been brought by a friend, and she generously offered Dr. Hauer a piece. Almost immediately she looked stricken, stating, "I told you the orderly took them. . .Oh no, why would I want to get him in trouble?!"

This case demonstrates two aspects of HIV-associated dementia: "misremembering" by merging of information, and the use of cueing to facilitate recall. Roberta experienced the orderly as rough, and she was later unable to locate her candy. She may then have thought that the orderly took it, and confirmed her own suspicions by remembering her feelings about the brusque treatment. When attention was called to the candy, this cued her memory.

Although Dr. Hauer was unable to conduct formal testing, Roberta's behavior and impaired memory suggested a diagnosis of possible HIV-associated dementia. Review of Roberta's medical condition, including blood tests, brain MRI, and current medications, excluded other causes of her behavioral symptoms. Further examination for depression did not reveal significant symptomatology. Dr. Hauer informed hospital staff of Roberta's diagnosis, and they structured her environment to reduce demands placed upon her. For example, they explained procedures before conducting them, confirming that she understood what was to take place. They kept clutter in her room to a minimum. They created a "memory book" so that she could record important information, events, and appointments.

Opportunistic Diseases

Summary

- Four HIV-related opportunistic conditions commonly cause cognitive impairment: toxoplasmosis, cryptococcal meningitis, progressive multifocal leukoencephalopathy, and lymphoma.
- Toxoplasmosis, a parasitic infection, may affect different parts of the brain and therefore cause different symptoms, ranging from motor weakness and sensory loss to seizures. Common presenting symptoms of toxoplasmosis include fever and constant headache. While the toxoplasma organism cannot be eliminated, toxoplasmosis symptoms can be controlled through drug treatment.
- Cryptococcal meningitis, a fungal infection, typically presents with fever and severe headache. Mental status changes range from mild behavioral and personality changes to severe memory loss and confusion. Antifungal drugs can clear infection.
- Progressive multifocal leukoencephalopathy (PML) is a neuropsychiatric disease caused by infection by the JC virus. Soon after infection, clients require major assistance with tasks of daily living and often become bed-bound. Death usually results within

several months. There are encouraging reports of a small number of clients who stabilize in response to experimental treatments.

- Other infections of the brain that cause impairment include: herpes, cytomegalovirus, CNS tuberculosis, and neurosyphilis.
- Lymphoma, a cancer originating in the lymphatic system, can invade the brain and cause cognitive impairment, behavioral and personality changes, and neurologic deficits. Radiation therapy is the most effective form of treatment for brain lymphoma.

Common HIV-related opportunistic infections and cancers of the central nervous system are a significant cause of cognitive impairment and, like other opportunistic infections, manifest when the immune system is significantly weakened. The nature of the particular tumor or pathogenic agent – parasite, virus, or fungus – as well as the location of the brain lesion it causes, will determine the pattern of symptoms in an individual client. This section describes the clinical manifestations of the main opportunistic infections and tumors that affect the brain, emphasizing the behavioral and cognitive abnormalities they can cause.[27]

Toxoplasmosis

Toxoplasma gondii, a parasite that is able to live within human cells, causes the most common HIV-related opportunistic infection of the brain. Toxoplasmosis (or "toxo" as it is colloquially called), the clinical disease that the organism produces, causes a number of neurologic symptoms, for example, muscle weakness, incoordination, and seizures, as well as transient mental status changes and sustained cognitive impairment. The organism is ubiquitous; studies suggest that 50 percent of people in the United States have been exposed to toxoplasma, but the parasite seldom causes clinically evident disease unless a person is immunologically compromised. Toxoplasmosis is the AIDS-defining diagnosis for approximately 5 percent of people with AIDS in the United States. HIV-infected immigrants from countries where exposure to *Toxoplasma gondii* is higher – for example, Haiti and France – have a higher incidence of toxoplasmosis.[28]

When the toxoplasma organism becomes active, it typically causes multiple infectious masses in different parts of the brain. This accounts for its varying clinical presentations; depending on the part of the brain that is infected, symptoms may include motor weakness, sensory loss, and focal seizures, that is, those limited to specific muscle groups. Common presenting symptoms of toxoplasmosis include fever and constant headache. Subtle changes in mental status – including confusion, memory loss, and ill-defined personality or behavior change – may predate presenting symptoms by weeks.

Diagnosis of toxoplasmosis is accomplished in three ways. Blood tests for antibodies to the organism document exposure, MRI of the brain reveals the characteristic pattern of multiple mass lesions, and analysis of cerebrospinal fluid (CSF) obtained by lumbar puncture ("spinal tap") rules out other infectious causes of symptoms.

Antibiotic therapy with sulfadiazine and pyrimethamine is effective in treating acute toxoplasmosis. However, since the organism is never eliminated, suppressive therapy with these antibiotics is necessary for the duration of the client's life to prevent active infection.

Cryptococcal Meningitis

Cryptococcus neoformans is the yeast-like fungus that causes cryptococcal meningitis, an infection of the outer covering of the brain (the meninges) seen in 5 percent to 10 percent of people with AIDS.[29] "Crypto," as it is commonly known, is the most common fungal infection of the brain in people with HIV disease. It typically presents with fever and severe headache, although initial symptoms may be more subtle with mild headache, nausea, and ill-defined malaise. Mental status changes may range from mild behavioral or personality changes to severe memory loss and confusion similar to that seen in HIV-associated dementia.

To accurately diagnose cryptococcal brain disease, clients must undergo lumbar puncture and CSF analysis. Several tests detect the presence of the fungus in the spinal fluid. Brain imaging with MRI or CT is generally not useful except to rule out other conditions, since cryptococcus rarely causes the mass lesions that would become apparent through these scans.

Effective treatment requires intravenous amphotericin B for six weeks. Following successful treatment, ongoing suppressive antifungal therapy with fluconazole should prevent relapse.

PML and Other Infections

Progressive multifocal leukoencephalopathy (PML) is a devastating neuropsychiatric disease caused by infection of the white matter of the brain with the JC virus. Approximately 2 percent of people with AIDS develop this condition, which can at times be difficult to differentiate from HIV-associated dementia.[30]

Following JC infection, PML develops quickly causing extensive damage to the myelin covering the nerves responsible for carrying motor signals to the muscles. Although the course of PML may be variable, with periods of decline alternating with periods of relative stability, usually clients require major assistance with tasks of daily living and often become bed-bound. Death usually results within several months, although there are encouraging reports of a small number of clients who stabilize in response to experimental treatment with very high dose zidovudine (ZDV; AZT) or with cytosine arabinoside administered into the cerebral-spinal fluid.

PML typically causes marked focal neurological symptoms, including hemiparesis (one-sided weakness), partial loss of vision, or impaired walking. It usually results in cognitive impairment with memory loss and visual-spatial dysfunction, and behavioral and personality changes as the illness progresses. In the presence of PML, MRI scan usually shows multiple abnormalities in the white matter areas of the brain. Single white matter lesions and JC infection of other parts of the brain occur occasionally.

Definitive diagnosis of PML is difficult to make without a brain biopsy. Instead, PML is most frequently diagnosed on the basis not only of cognitive impairment but also of marked focal neurological symptoms, which are not present in HIV-associated dementia. MRI scans are necessary to rule out other opportunistic conditions and confirm the pathologic changes in the white matter.

Although not as common as toxoplasmosis, cryptococcal meningitis, and PML, there are other infectious agents that invade the brain and cause cognitive impairment and neurological symptoms in clients with AIDS. These include:

- *Herpes simplex I and II:* the viruses that cause oral, anal, and genital ulcers;
- *Herpes zoster:* the virus that causes "shingles";
- *Cytomegalovirus (CMV):* the virus that infects the retina, causing blindness;
- *Mycobacterium tuberculosis:* the same organism responsible for pulmonary tuberculosis, often presenting with cranial nerve weakness;

- *Treponema pallidum:* the cause of syphilis, which can remain latent in the body for years before causing symptoms of dementia and neurological impairment in its late stages.

Brain (CNS) Lymphoma

Lymphoma, a cancer originating in the lymphatic system, is a common complication of AIDS. In approximately 7 percent of AIDS patients, lymphoma invades the brain causing clinical symptoms, including cognitive impairment, behavioral and personality changes, and neurologic deficits.[31]

Some clients with brain lymphoma may appear similar to those with HIV-associated dementia, but the presence of significant focal neurologic symptoms, for example, one-sided weakness, often differentiates the two conditions. CT or MRI scans are critical to the diagnosis of CNS lymphoma, although at times a brain biopsy may be necessary to confirm the cancer and distinguish the case from toxoplasmosis. Radiation therapy is the most effective form of treatment for brain lymphoma and it has been shown to prolong life in patients with AIDS by shrinking tumor size; even with treatment, however, life expectancy is only six months after diagnosis.

PML and Progressive Disability: The Case of Derek

Derek was a 26-year-old gay man, reportedly seronegative, brought to the hospital emergency room by his lover Jerry. Jerry was alarmed about Derek's increasing confusion and memory loss, which had emerged over the prior two months. Derek had appeared to be healthy, working as a paralegal until three months earlier when he had decided to quit because of low energy and difficulty concentrating. Jerry noticed a gradual increase in social withdrawal.

When Derek did get up and walk around, his movements were notably slower and more deliberate. He would occasionally stumble and hold on to furniture for support. In recent weeks, Derek began having trouble remembering what day it was or following simple instructions; he also acted strangely, for example, he would put dirty dishes in the refrigerator, not the dishwasher. His speaking ability was reduced, and he answered most questions simply "yes" or "no."

Upon presentation at the hospital emergency room, Derek underwent a brief medical evaluation, which found no obvious cause for his symptoms. He appeared physically healthy, but because he continued to show dramatic changes in mental status and ability to care for himself, he was admitted to the inpatient psychiatry unit for a full evaluation under the care of Louise Goldwyn, MD. Antibody testing was positive, and a T-helper cell count of 20 indicated profound immune suppression and a diagnosis of AIDS. MRI brain scan showed shrinkage of brain tissue (atrophy) and demyelinating lesions of the white matter consistent with a diagnosis of PML. Neurological examination showed significant muscle weakness and incoordination. Nursing staff reported episodic bladder incontinence.

Dr. Goldwyn initiated treatment with ZDV in an attempt to slow PML progression. Nursing staff planned a routine of care that emphasized consistency and simplicity. They placed large signs on the ward with arrows indicating directions to Derek's room and the bathroom. This planning allowed Derek to accept the nursing assistance even when he did not seem to understand what was happening to him.

Dr. Goldwyn and John Farmer, Derek's social worker, held a series of meetings with Jerry and Derek's extended family of origin. They discussed PML and the likelihood that Derek would soon become even more disabled. After several meetings, it was decided that Derek would live at his parents' home with in-home nursing care. Shortly thereafter, however, Derek's rapidly progressing disability required his transfer to a hospital unit that specialized in the care of patients with HIV-associated cognitive impairment. In the course of these meetings, it became clear that Jerry was also in considerable distress, and Mr. Farmer referred him to a weekly support group for partners and family members of people with dementia.

In the weeks before transfer to the specialized dementia care unit, Derek continued to lose both strength and cognitive ability. He required increasing assistance from nursing staff with basic functioning. By the time of his transfer, he was bed-bound and mute. He died shortly after the transfer.

Organic Affective Disorders

Summary

- "Organic affective disorders" are disturbances of mood that result from specific and known biological causes, such as a viral infection, a stroke, a tumor, long-term substance abuse, or dementia. The two most common disorders are mania and depression.

- Organic mania is characterized by an elated or irritable mood, and by behavior demonstrating at least two of the following features: hyperactivity, pressured speech, flight of ideas, grandiosity, decreased sleep, distractibility, and lack of judgment. It causes transient symptoms that interfere with abilities to reason, problem-solve, and be attentive, and often occurs concurrently with impairment caused by direct HIV infection of the brain.
- Organic depression is characterized by persistent feelings of saddened mood and loss of interest or pleasure in nearly all activities. These symptoms may lead to impaired attention and concentration, and mimic or co-exist with other cognitive changes.

Organic "affective disorders," also known as "mood disorders," are disturbances of mood that result from specific and known biological causes such as viral infection, stroke, tumor, chronic substance abuse, or dementia. These organic affective disorders typically take the form of either depression or mania and are often accompanied by cognitive impairment or dementia. Organic mood syndromes are particularly common in subcortical disorders like HIV-associated dementia, Parkinson's Disease, and Huntington's Disease.[32]

Among patients with HIV infection, the risk of an organic affective disorder increases as immune suppression increases. These disorders, particularly mania, often occur concurrently with HIV-associated minor cognitive/motor disorder and may herald the development of HIV-associated dementia. However, they are more typically associated with moderate to severe HIV-associated cognitive impairment, that is, dementia itself.[26]

Diagnosis of mood disorders requires a good psychiatric history including substance use and family history, level of immunosuppression, and current medication regimen. It is crucial to be aware of conditions and vulnerabilities specific to HIV disease in order to rule out delirium, neuropsychiatric disorders secondary to opportunistic illnesses or lymphoma, and drug reactions.

Organic Mania

Organic mania, similar in its symptoms to the mania of bipolar disorder, is a psychiatric disorder resulting from medical, pharmacological, or other organic dysfunction lasting at least one week. It is characterized by an elated or irritable mood and by behavior demonstrating at least two of the following features: hyperactivity, pressured speech, flight of ideas, grandiosity, decreased sleep, distractibility, and lack of judgment.[33] Grandiose delusions, irritability, and euphoria are particularly common.[34] Even after treatment, residual distractibility and poor judgment, if not more significant cognitive impairment, may be evident.[35]

Organic mania differs in origin from bipolar mania, which is a primary psychiatric condition; the major distinction between the two is that bipolar mania is not caused by any known medical condition and is usually related to a history of mania among family members. In fact, a family history of manic depressive or other affective disease, or the coexistence of the manic syndrome with confusional states[33] – which indicate delirium – are criteria for excluding a diagnosis of HIV-related mania.

In addition to causing symptoms of cognitive impairment in and of itself, organic mania has been increasingly associated with cognitive impairment caused by direct HIV infection of the brain.[3,36,37] The relationship between the two remains unclear: is mania an aspect of HIV-associated dementia, or are the two discrete but associated disorders?[34]

It has been hypothesized that HIV-associated mania is a presenting feature in the triad of cognitive, motor, and behavioral symptoms connected with both HIV-associated minor cognitive/motor disorder and HIV-associated dementia. For example, in one case study, psychotherapists considered eight patients to be cognitively intact prior to psychotic manic episodes, but neuropsychological deficits were revealed once psychotic symptoms abated.[35] A review of HIV-related psychiatric studies suggests that among AIDS patients, organic mania may be a precursor to a rapid decline toward severe dementia or death.[38]

An early study estimated the incidence of HIV-related mania as 16 percent to 20 percent among patients with HIV-associated dementia.[3] A more recent study estimates that people with HIV disease face a fourfold increase in risk of mania when compared to the general population.[35] It is important to note that an organic manic episode may also be associated with medications including steroids, antidepressants, and in rare instances ZDV, as well as with amphetamine or cocaine use. Clinicians should consider these alternative causes prior to treating mania as if it were HIV-related.

Depression

Depression is characterized by persistent feelings of sadness and loss of interest or pleasure in nearly all activities. Additional symptoms may include: changes in appetite or weight; changes in sleep and psychomotor activity (agitation or slowing); decreased energy; feelings of worthlessness or guilt; and recurrent thoughts of death or suicide. Depression may also lead to cognitive changes, including impaired attention and concentration, slowed thinking, and apparent memory loss.

Depression is common among both HIV-infected and uninfected people, particularly those seeking psychotherapy. Since HIV is known to infect subcortical brain structures – thought to be the sites of mood regulation[32] – it may be reasonably postulated that some cases of depression are organic, that is, due to direct HIV infection.

HIV-related organic depression emerges later in the course of HIV disease as immunosuppression increases, and it may respond less well to antidepressant medication than other forms of depression. Clinically, the cause of depression in HIV-infected patients may be a moot point, because despite this caveat, major depression and HIV-related organic depression are treated similarly. In addition, depression is difficult to diagnose in HIV-infected patients for two reasons: symptoms of HIV disease, for example, weight loss, resemble the physical or somatic symptoms of depression; and the apathy and social withdrawal seen in patients with HIV-associated dementia resembles that seen in people with depression.

Neuropsychological assessment is the best method for identifying and differentiating depression from cognitive impairment caused by other conditions. When it is not available, however, a good history and neuropsychiatric interview are helpful. Consider the following:

- Physical symptoms such as loss of appetite, weight loss, and sleep disturbance may be due to HIV infection rather than depression. Focus instead on sadness, decreased ability to experience pleasure, feelings of worthlessness, and suicidal ideation related to a sense of failure.[9]
- In asymptomatic HIV-infected individuals, self-report of cognitive changes such as memory impairment is infrequent and is primarily associated with depression.[39] In symptomatic or immunosuppressed individuals, self-report of these changes

should raise suspicion of cognitive impairment.

- Patients with dementia tend to look apathetic and affectively flat, but lack the sadness or distress seen in depression.
- Prior depressive episodes and a family history of depression increase the risk of depression.
- HIV-related medications – including ZDV and trimethoprim/sulfamethoxazole (Septra or Bactrim) – may contribute to depression.
- Depression may be related to alcohol or substance use.
- Depression and HIV-related cognitive impairment may co-exist.

Clinicians should maintain a low threshold for treatment of depression. That is, they should err on the side of treatment, since current antidepressant medications have fewer side effects and are less risky than older ones. It is important to note that once depression is effectively treated, an underlying cognitive impairment, related to another cause, may become evident.

Mania and Grandiose Behavior: The Case of Ralph

Ralph, a 29-year-old bisexual man and former substance user, was involuntarily admitted to a locked psychiatric unit after speeding down the highway and failing to stop for police sirens. He told hospital staff that he had rubbed his car with olive oil and peanut butter "to make it invisible to law enforcement,"

On admission, Ralph was intrusive and animated to the point of agitation. His gait was clumsy, and his speech was pressured. He exhibited loose associations, flight of ideas, and grandiose delusional thinking: for example, he said, "30,000 people from Las Vegas are coming to my birthday party." He was emotionally labile, fluctuating between irritability and euphoria. The admitting psychiatrist, Susan Powell, diagnosed manic psychosis.

A history gathered from Ralph's roommate, Phil, was notable in terms of three facts: Ralph was HIV-infected, he had exhibited increasing behavioral disorganization over the prior month, and he had not used drugs for two years. A drug toxicity screen confirmed this.

Neuropsychological testing indicated moderate to severe HIV-associated dementia with motor and cognitive slowing, severe memory deficit, cognitive rigidity, visual-spatial impairment, and the inability to think abstractly. Results of laboratory tests and CSF examination were normal. However, an MRI brain scan showed diffuse white matter disease with generalized atrophy, consistent with HIV-associated dementia.

Ralph was initially treated with a mood stabilizer, divalproex sodium, and an antipsychotic, perphenazine. After five days, Ralph's agitation and irritability diminished, although he continued to express mild euphoria and occasional references to invisibility. After increasing the Depakote over the next ten days, Ralph's mood normalized, and he was able to focus on plans to move to his parents' home.

Transient Impairment

Summary

- Organic conditions such as delirium and substance intoxication cause short-lived and reversible cognitive impairment.
- Delirium – frequently called "a confusional state" – is a syndrome, a combination of cognitive and behavioral symptoms that includes alteration of consciousness, confusion, and memory loss, and which may lead to death.
- Substance abuse can lead to acute episodes of psychosis, including confusion, agitation, or manic symptoms.

Some cognitive impairment is "transient," that is, short-lived and reversible. Transient impairment is due to identifiable organic causes. The most common causes among HIV-infected clients are delirium and substance intoxication. The existence of one of these conditions, however, does not rule out the possibility of permanent, stable cognitive impairment caused by other conditions that may become evident after the transient state subsides.

Delirium

Delirium – frequently called "a confusional state" – is a common medical syndrome of transient brain dysfunction causing reversible cognitive impairment, a disturbance of consciousness, and other brain-related symptoms. Delirium is a syndrome, with a variety of symptoms and underlying causes, many of which have life-threatening effects on organ systems, including the brain. (See Table 2: Potential Causes of Delirium in HIV Disease, page 27.) For example, low serum sodium may result in delirium leading to seizures and death. Symptoms of delirium include confusion and memory loss and may be mistakenly attributed to either HIV-associated minor

Table 2. Potential Causes of Delirium in HIV Disease[40]

Central Nervous System Opportunists
- Toxoplasmosis
- Cryptococcal meningitis
- Herpes encephalitis
- Neurosyphilis
- Cytomegalovirus encephalitis
- Progressive multifocal leukoencephalopathy
- Brain lymphoma

Antibiotic Medications
- Ciprofloxacin
- Metronidazole (Flagyl)

Other Medications Used in HIV Disease
- Antiemetics: Dronabinol (Marinol)
- Antihistamines: diphenhydramine (Benadryl) and others
- Glucocorticoids: prednisone (Deltasone) and others
- Opiate pain medications:
  - morphine (Roxanol), oxycodone (Percodan) and others

Psychiatric Medications
- Antidepressants: amitryptyline (Elavil), doxepin (Sinequan), and others
- Antiparkinsonians: benztropine (Cogentin) and others
- Antipsychotics: haloperidol (Haldol), thioridazine (Mellaril), and others
- Benzodiazepines: triazolam (Halcion), diazepam (Valium), and others

cognitive/motor disorder or HIV-associated dementia. Early recognition of delirium is critical to allow for prompt treatment, and to provide the best chance of recovery from this often fatal condition.

Delirium typically develops over a relatively brief time course – from hours to days – although it can evolve more slowly. Abrupt changes in mental status, particularly in the level of consciousness, are signs of delirium. Patients may present in either a highly aroused, hyperactive state or in a withdrawn, immobile condition. Symptoms often worsen as daylight wanes and patients misinterpret environmental stimuli; a patient, coherent in the morning, may appear disoriented in the evening. Because of this fluctuation, "serial" mental status examinations, conducted several times daily and over consecutive days, are necessary to accurately assess delirium.

Orientation, attention and concentration, and ability to learn new material are the most likely functions to be impaired in the presence of delirium. Accompanying symptoms may include auditory and visual hallucinations, delusions, disorganized speech, muteness, and irritability. Repetitive motor behaviors, for example, purposeless picking at clothing or sheets, are suggestive of delirium, as is tremulousness and other new-onset, abnormal movements. In response to suspicions that delirium is present, clinicians should undertake aggressive efforts to identify and treat underlying causes at the same time as they treat specific behavioral symptoms.

HIV-related delirium has many causes, including the opportunistic infections and neoplasms discussed above. In addition, many therapeutic agents used by people with HIV disease can cause delirium.[40] The larger the number of medications that an individual takes, the greater the likelihood of harmful interactions like delirium. Psychiatric medications, for example, benzodiazepines or the anticholinergic effects of some antidepressants and antipsychotics, may cause changes in mentation. Drugs of abuse may also cause delirium, both through the effects of intoxication and delayed withdrawal.

The systemic effects of HIV disease frequently lead to delirious states with symptoms of cognitive impairment. These systemic conditions include electrolyte imbalance and toxic metabolic states due to organ failure or disseminated infection of the blood (sepsis) by bacteria, virus, or fungus. People with HIV disease are also susceptible to a variety of syndromes that reduce the flow of blood and oxygen to the brain, interrupting brain function and causing cognitive impairment and other symptoms of delirium. Anemia (low red blood cell count), hypoxia (lack of oxygen entering the blood via the lungs due to pneumonia or other complications), and dehydration leading to reduced blood volume are all frequent effects of HIV disease that may cause delirium.

Dosage and Delirium: The Case of Gabriel

Gabriel is a 34-year-old Latino gay man with AIDS who entered psychotherapy with Louis Tanaka, LCSW for help with feelings of depression and anxiety related to his advancing HIV disease. Gabriel continued to work as a plumber in his own business, but became increasingly aware of his physical limitations. He was troubled by painful neuropathy in his lower legs and shortness of breath due to a prior episode of *Pneumocystis carinii* pneumonia.

Mr. Tanaka helped Gabriel explore his fears of what would happen as he became increasingly disabled. Gabriel was able to consider ways of asking others for help, something that had previously felt unacceptable. As psychotherapy progressed, Gabriel's mood gradually improved and he was able to cope more effectively with daily stresses. Improvement continued steadily until one session when Mr. Tanaka noted a dramatic change.

Gabriel was lethargic, occasionally staring off at nothing in particular. His thinking was disorganized and he repeatedly referred to his employees, accusing them of embezzling money from him, and he threatened to call the police. Mr. Tanaka inquired about new stresses or medical problems, but Gabriel denied any changes, saying instead, "Those workers are stealing me blind."

Still concerned about the acute change in mental status, Mr. Tanaka phoned Rhonda Newell, MD, Gabriel's physician at the AIDS Clinic, to see if she had noticed similar changes. Dr. Newell was surprised, having seen Gabriel in her office the previous week and having found him to be his usual self. However, she did report that she had prescribed two new medications to treat the pain associated with his worsening neuropathy. Both medications, amitriptyline (Elavil) and acetaminophen with codeine (TyCo #3) are known to cause mental status changes, especially in medically ill patients .

Mr. Tanaka urged Gabriel to go to Dr. Newell's office for an examination and blood work. Her evaluation showed no signs of opportunistic infections, and Dr. Newell made a diagnosis of delirium caused by the anticholinergic effect of the amitriptyline and the opiate effect of the codeine. She discontinued the medications, and Gabriel gradually returned to his usual mental state over the next several days. Mr. Tanaka assisted Gabriel in arranging for friends to stay with him at home during the recovery period. When Gabriel's pain recurred, Dr. Newell prescribed a lower dose of codeine, which provided adequate relief without leading to delirium.

Substance Abuse

Substance abuse is most likely to cause transient symptoms of cognitive impairment, although chronic heavy use may also be associated with more permanent symptoms. The transient symptoms associated with acute use and withdrawal vary with the substance used and may include impaired attention, memory loss, and disorientation.

Since these symptoms can mimic both psychiatric and organic disorders, substance abuse-related impairment can be difficult to diagnose. For example, an individual abusing cocaine or amphetamines may present with an acute episode of psychosis, including confusion, agitation, or manic symptoms. Substance abuse may also result in a secondary psychiatric disorder and related cognitive impairment. For instance, chronic use of alcohol, amphetamines, or cocaine can cause depression and problems with concentration and memory.

In some cases, substance abuse may be associated with permanent cognitive impairment that may predate HIV infection. Regardless of HIV-infection status, injection drug use is statistically correlated with an increased incidence of learning disabilities, educational failure, and head injury with resulting diminished performance on neuropsychological testing. Correspondingly, HIV-infected injection drug users tend to perform more poorly on neuropsychological testing than HIV-infected people who do not use these drugs.[41] Substance abuse may lead to permanent deficits in attention and memory. As a result, among substance users, motor abnormalities may be the first clear sign of HIV-associated minor cognitive/motor disorder.[18,42]

The complicated question of triple diagnosis – distinguishing depression from cognitive impairment from substance abuse – is common in HIV-associated psychiatry. When faced with this diagnostic question, it is helpful to define the level of immunosuppression. In general, the higher the T-helper cell count, the less likely it is that there is HIV-related cognitive impairment. At this point, providers should focus on delineating between a psychiatric disorder and a substance-induced disorder.

The medical work-up for substance abuse consists of a thorough drug and psychiatric history, a urine toxicology screen for the presence of drugs, and a physical examination, which may reveal needle marks. In the hospital setting, staff are trained to look for withdrawal symptoms, which vary depending on the substance used, and for rapid clearing of cognitive impairment and behavioral disturbance. The use of stimulants, however, can result in a psychotic disorder that can last weeks after last use, and prolonged paranoid delusions may complicate assessment of underlying cognitive impairment.[43]

2

Diagnostic Evaluation

CAREFUL diagnosis is crucial to distinguish among the variety of conditions that cause cognitive impairment and determine appropriate prognosis and treatment.[44] The diagnostic process begins with a mental status examination and neuropsychiatric interview to assess presenting symptoms and overall level of neuropsychiatric functioning. These procedures may be conducted by a psychotherapist or primary health care provider. If this evaluation suggests cognitive impairment or neuropsychiatric disturbance, the front-line provider may wish to refer the client to a psychiatric social worker, psychologist, or psychiatrist familiar with HIV disease for a neuropsychiatric interview to corroborate the initial diagnostic impression of impairment. Neurologic examination and laboratory and radiologic testing are critical to clarify the specific cause of impairment. These examinations are best performed by physicians or nurse practitioners who are familiar with HIV disease, HIV-related opportunistic conditions, and delirious states that may cause cognitive impairment. If the diagnostic picture remains unclear, it may be necessary for a neuropsychologist to undertake neuropsychological testing, a more detailed and specific assessment of cognitive and other functional abilities.

Summary

- Diagnosis of causes of HIV-related cognitive impairment is complicated because symptoms may vary minimally across disorders. Treatment, however, varies dramatically and so accurate diagnosis is crucial. There are five procedures used in diagnosis: mental status examination, neuropsychiatric interview, neurologic examination, laboratory and radiologic testing, and neuropsychological testing.
- A mental status examination aims at detecting deficits in basic cognitive functions by looking at a variety of indicators including: general appearance, motor coordination, memory, language, affect, orientation, and concentration.
- A neuropsychiatric interview expands upon the mental status examination, adding a comprehensive medical and psychological history.
- A neurologic examination focuses on specific indicators of neurological functioning including walking, coordination, and muscle tone.
- There are a range of laboratory and radiologic tests that can act as adjuncts to more clinical approaches. These tests provide chemical and biological indicators that can help distinguish among the variety of causes of cognitive impairment.
- Neuropsychological testing uses standardized measures, primarily paper-and-pencil tests, to assess cognitive, behavioral, and emotional indicators of suspected brain dysfunction that may not become evident through other procedures.

Mental Status Examination

A mental status exam is designed to test a variety of mental functions that may be altered by neuropsychiatric disorders.[44] It includes observation of appearance and behavior, and active evaluation through questions and answers of specific cognitive functions.

Although there is some overlap among the parts of the exam, for example, attention is necessary for memory, each part aims to assess a separate area of cognitive functioning. The pattern of performance on the exam can be helpful in distinguishing among the causes of impairment, particularly in diagnosing disorders such as delirium or depression. Although most psychotherapists will not undertake a formal mental status exam, looking for cognitive, behavioral, and motor changes over time can uncover impairment as it develops and lead to appropriate referral and treatment. Regular charting of progress notes can be helpful in tracking such changes.

General Appearance: Note hygiene and grooming for cleanliness, disarrangement, and the use of appropriate clothing. Clients with advanced AIDS may be emaciated, sometimes noted in medical charts as "cachectic," with prominent facial bones and sunken eyes. This is a sign of late-stage AIDS when there is increased likelihood of cognitive impairment.

Motor Behavior: Look for slowness, weakness, and gait disturbance. In contrast, clients with organic mania may be agitated and hyperactive. Fine motor incoordination may be a first symptom of HIV-associated dementia. An easily observed sign of motor incoordination is a change in handwriting on checks offered in payment for psychotherapy.

Language: Speech may be preserved even with moderate cognitive impairment, but language may indicate subtle changes. Look for slowed speech, decreased spontaneity and initiation, lag in response time, and a paucity of content.

Thought Process: Rambling speech is often evident with HIV-associated dementia. Clients may get stuck on a topic and may have difficulty shifting when the subject is changed. In attempting to carry out a complex task, they may lose track of steps or may compensate by self-cueing, that is, talking themselves through a task as they perform it step-by-step. While these changes may not be so evident in therapy, clients or family members may be able to describe problem-solving difficulties especially in new situations or with new tasks.

Thought Content: As impairment progresses, clients tend to focus more and more on the past. With HIV-related mania, they may describe paranoid and grandiose delusions.

Affect: Affect gradually becomes blunted, and clients may appear apathetic or indifferent. Unlike depressed clients, who express despair or unhappiness, clients with HIV-associated dementia appear flat or seem emotionally absent. Manic clients may present as irritable or euphoric.

Level of Consciousness ("Sensorium"): Clients are generally alert until end stage AIDS. Consider delirium if there is a fluctuating level of consciousness, and refer for evaluation for an acute brain disorder such as delirium or toxoplasmosis.

Orientation: Clients are usually oriented to person, place, and date until late in the course of HIV-associated dementia. At that point, they may be unable to remember dates and may become confused about the location.

Attention and Concentration: The ability to perform simple tasks such as repeating digits is generally preserved until late in the course of HIV disease. A traditional mental status exam uses multi-step tasks to look for lapses in concentration: spelling "world" backwards, performing serial sevens (serial subtraction of seven from 100), giving a three-step command, or performing calculations. In psychotherapy, concentration may be assessed by asking the client questions that require computation, for example, "How old were you when ——?"

Memory: Immediate memory is usually preserved in HIV-associated minor cognitive/motor disorder, and clients are able to repeat a short list of words after five minutes. A delay of twenty to thirty minutes is necessary to uncover memory impairment. After such a delay, clients with moderate impairment may not spontaneously recall information. A clue or prompt, however, may help them remember. In later stages of HIV-associated dementia, memory impairment becomes more severe and is observable even after a short delay. In psychotherapy, clients may describe episodes of memory impairment, repeat information from previous sessions or from earlier in the hour, or begin to miss appointments.

Visual-Spatial Information: Visual-spatial memory impairment is particularly evident in HIV-associated dementia and may lead to a variety of symptoms including getting lost or confused in familiar settings. Visual-spatial memory can be tested by asking the client to copy a geometric design and then reproduce it 20 to 30 minutes later. This is a good task for distinguishing depression from dementia, because demented people have diminished recall (people with normal cognitive function remember at least 70 percent). In addition, the geometric designs rendered from memory by demented patients tends to be simplified and of poor quality.

Abstraction: Mental status exams usually include a measure of abstraction to test the ability to conceptualize and manipulate less concrete information. In early or moderate stages of HIV-related cognitive impairment, however, these measures are not particularly sensitive or useful.

Insight and Judgment: Insight and judgment, as exemplified by awareness of deficits, varies widely among clients with HIV-related cognitive impairment, and formal testing often will not detect such limitations. Hypothetical questions may lead to simple, abbreviated answers, but when asked to elaborate, people with HIV-associated dementia will often give correct responses. On the other hand, comparisons to client history may offer a good way to evaluate recent changes in judgment. It may also be useful to ask personal questions like, "What are your plans for the next week?", and if appropriate, "What are your plans after you leave the hospital?"

Neuropsychiatric Interview

A neuropsychiatric interview – consisting of a careful history of recent and present symptoms as recounted by the client, in addition to a mental status exam[45] – provides a measure of current neurobehavioral status. For mental health providers seeing HIV-infected clients over time, this evaluation can be adapted and performed on a periodic basis, creating a baseline for future comparisons and tracking a drop in function.

The focus of the interview should be the client's current ability to function at work and in activities of daily living. To establish an estimate of usual functioning, ask about education and occupation. This information can help establish what skills should be well-honed and clarify decrements in functioning.

If possible, interview the client both alone and in the presence of a partner, friend, or family member. This may facilitate a more accurate portrayal of cognitive difficulties, since clients may be experiencing memory loss, apathy, or psychological or organic denial about their deficits.

Ask about past and present medical and psychiatric illnesses or symptoms. Be alert that a T-helper cell count of less than 200 or the presence of other AIDS-defining illnesses increases the risk of HIV-related cognitive impairment.

Ask specifically about any recent changes at work or in daily life, if the client has needed help with tasks or has ceased any work or social activities. Sometimes asking the client to describe an average day can elicit this information. Consider in particular the following potential deficits:

- Changes in motor function, including handwriting, balance, walking;
- Decreased ability to concentrate, including difficulty following conversations, difficulty following the plot of a book or television show;
- Memory loss, including forgetting appointments or conversations, or getting lost;
- Emotional changes, including increased irritability or emotional lability;
- Decreased ability to do complex tasks, including managing money, planning or cooking meals, or fulfilling work demands.

A number of studies have correlated complaints of behavioral and cognitive changes, in particular motor symptoms, with neuropsychological performance.[46,47,48,49] Some symptoms, however, are associated with depression and clinicians must rule out this condition before diagnosing HIV-related cognitive impairment.[39] Motor symptoms and performance on a mental status exam may indicate organic HIV-related cognitive impairment, but differentiation may require more sensitive neuropsychological testing.

Neurologic Examination

A neurologic examination focuses on specific indicators of neurological functioning in order to uncover the neurological deficits that signify central nervous system disease, including acute brain disorders like toxoplasmosis, and progressive disorders like HIV-associated dementia and PML. Neurological examinations are typically performed by a client's primary doctor or nurse practitioner, however, a neurologist may be called in for a specialty consultation.

There are several indicators of impaired neurological functioning:

Walking: Walking may reveal slowness, leg weakness, and unsteady gait.

Coordination: Several tests measure lack of coordination, including: rapid alternating movement testing, whereby the client is asked to repetitively and alternately clench one fist while at the same time opening wide the other hand; and the finger-nose test, whereby the client touches the examiner's finger (which is held several inches in front of the client's face), his or her own nose, and again the examiner's finger, repeating these movements back and forth, sometimes with the examiner's finger stationary and sometimes with it moving.

Muscle Tone: Eventually, in addition to general weakness, there is likely to be abnormally heightened muscle tone, increased to the point of stiffness. When reflexes are tested by tapping on the knee tendon, the client displays hyper-reflexia, the muscle response is increased, and the leg jerks up further than usual. This is seen equally on both sides of the body. Other reflexes, called frontal release signs – including the grasp reflex – are present in healthy infants, but abnormal in adults. When seen in adults, they indicate significant brain disease and are frequently seen in clients with dementia.

Laboratory and Radiologic Testing

The following tests are important adjuncts in evaluating HIV-related cognitive impairment. Blood tests are routine and done in virtually all patients who are being assessed. Brain scans (either MRI or CT) should be included as part of the evaluation but are not always readily available due to cost. Lumbar puncture is not done routinely but may be important in some clinical situations, for example, to rule out neurosyphilis.

T-Helper Cell Count: Also called "CD4+," the T-helper cell is a white blood cell crucial to immunity. Its level generally indicates the strength of the immune system. HIV-associated dementia and opportunistic diseases that impair cognition are unlikely when the T-helper counts are greater than 200. A normal count ranges from 420 to 1200, although it is important to note that the range used varies somewhat from laboratory to laboratory, and that counts can vary from time to time for the same individual.

Complete Blood Count: The complete blood count (CBC) provides total counts of white blood cells (WBC), red blood cells (RBC), and platelets. A low WBC suggests immune compromise, while a high WBC may indicate bacterial infection. A low RBC count indicates anemia, which may be caused by chronic infection, poor nutrition, chronic bleeding, or medications like ZDV. Very low platelet counts (less than 25,000/mm^3) predispose to bruising and bleeding.

Vitamin B_{12} and Folate: Abnormally low levels of these dietary elements in the blood can cause anemia, and cognitive and behavioral changes. Impaired absorption in the intestinal tract, which often occurs during HIV infection, can lower levels even when the diet is adequate.

Blood Chemistry: A panel of chemistry tests – including levels of electrolytes such as sodium and potassium, kidney functions, and liver functions – is useful in assessing the major organ systems of the body.

Thyroid Function Tests: Thyroid function tests (TFT) measure thyroid hormone in the blood, assessing low (hypothyroid) or high (hyperthyroid) thyroid levels, both of which can cause cognitive impairment and other mental status changes including mood disturbance and psychosis.

Syphilis Testing: Screening for syphilis – using VDRL, RPR, or MHA-TP screens – is important because in later stages, it infects the brain and can cause a dementia syndrome with mood and behavioral symptoms.

Cryptococcal Antigen: Detects cryptococcal antigen (CrAg) in the blood, which suggests the possibility of this fungal infection in the brain or in other parts of the body.

Toxoplasma Titer: Measures antibodies to *Toxoplasma gondii,* which suggests the possibility of toxoplasmosis infection of the brain.

Lumbar Puncture: Lumbar puncture (spinal tap) may be used to assess for an acute brain infection or other CNS opportunistic illness. To perform this procedure, cerebrospinal fluid is drawn through a needle, which is inserted into the lower back. CSF analysis will indicate infection, but will be generally normal or only slightly abnormal in cases of HIV-associated dementia.

Magnetic Resonance Imaging or Computerized Tomography: MRI scans demonstrate cerebral atrophy (decreased brain size) and white matter disease (patchy abnormalities in the myelin that connects different parts of the brain), but may be completely normal in some individuals with HIV-associated dementia. Although not as sensitive as MRI, CT scans show similar changes.

Electroencephalogram: Electroencephalograms (EEG) record electrical activity in the brain and can be abnormal in up to 40 percent of individuals with HIV-associated dementia. However, they are most useful in identifying seizure disorders that can accompany CNS opportunistic diseases.

Neuropsychological Testing

Neuropsychological testing uses standardized measures, primarily paper-and-pencil tests, to assess cognitive, behavioral, and emotional indicators of suspected brain dysfunction.[50] In clients with HIV disease, neuropsychological testing[18] is useful in the following instances:

- Detecting subtle signs of early brain disorder when the results of neurological, laboratory, and neuroimaging tests remain normal;
- Characterizing the nature and severity of the brain disorder based on pattern of performance;
- Assessing a related or separate psychiatric condition, such as depression;
- Providing a baseline measure to track potential cognitive decline;
- Planning treatment, the ability to work, or the level of care needed.

Neuropsychological testing is conducted by a neuropsychologist, a clinical psychologist with training in neuropsychology and preferably experience with HIV disease. The testing procedure consists of a clinical interview of the client and other people, for example, a partner, family member, or physician. The test battery assesses a general range of cognitive function at the same time as it targets a pattern of deficits specific to HIV-related cognitive impairment. In addition, personality tests may be used to assess anxiety and depression. To determine the presence, pattern, and degree of impairment, performance is compared with test norms of age- and education-matched people without brain dysfunction.

Symptomatic HIV-infected clients fatigue easily, so the test battery should be relatively short and focused. On the other hand, brief neuropsychiatric screening measures such as the Mini-Mental Status Exam are relatively insensitive to the cognitive deficits in HIV-infected clients and thus are not clinically useful. The battery chosen should provide information regarding an estimated preexisting level of cognitive functioning, attention, concentration, fine-motor speed, memory, visual-spatial ability, verbal fluency, problem-solving skills, mental speed, and information processing. The battery might include the following tests: The Shipley Institute of Living Scale[51]; Finger Tapping Test[52]; Strength of Grip[52]; Digit Span and Digit Symbol[53]; Buschke Selective Reminding Test[54]; Wechsler Memory Scale-Russell Revision[55]; Controlled Oral Word Association Test[50]; Trail Making Test[52]; and Short Booklet Category Test.[56]

It is important to note the limitations to neuropsychological testing.[57] First, it does not fully control for cultural variables and language barriers. In an attempt to address this shortcoming, the World Health Organization has developed a test battery for assessing HIV-infected non-English speaking people in other countries.[12] Although it is still being validated, this battery holds promise for testing monolingual non-English speakers in the United States. Second, clients must be cooperative and have the stamina for an evaluation that usually takes three to six hours (although this may be broken up into several days). Finally, neuropsychological testing generally costs between $600 and $1200, which may or may not be fully covered by health insurance.

Accurate Diagnosis and Appropriate Treatment

The diagnostic battery available to detect cognitive impairment matches in complexity the range of conditions that can cause impairment. This complexity may be daunting, but it is important to remember that diagnostic approaches are tools, that no single provider need understand the intricacies of all of these tools, and that psychiatrists, neurologists, and neuropsychologists can be useful resources in negotiating this diagnostic process. Most importantly, it is crucial to remember that many of these conditions are manageable and that accurate diagnosis can lead to appropriate treatment.

3

Treating and Managing Cognitive Impairment

SINCE mental health providers working with people with HIV disease frequently have more contact than other health professionals with these clients, they may be the first to notice cognitive, behavioral, or motor changes. Regardless of whether or not providers refer these clients for formal neuropsychiatric evaluation, they will continue to face concerns about cognitive impairment and how to manage it.

The goals of management are two-fold: to treat aggressively the acute causes of cognitive impairment, such as opportunistic infections and delirium; and to attenuate through psychopharmacology and psychotherapy the effects of organic affective disorders and the ongoing and progressive impairment caused by HIV infection of the brain. In order to accomplish these tasks, therapists need to alter the focus and technique of psychotherapy depending on the severity and course of impairment and the resulting interference with daily living.[57] They must also assume a larger role in coordinating care with physicians and consulting with family and friends who act as caregivers.

This chapter provides an overview of the management of HIV-related cognitive disorders, focusing on psychotherapeutic approaches, environmental or behavioral interventions, and psychopharmacological treatment. (For a discussion of medical treatment of opportunistic conditions and delirium, see Chapter 1 of the monograph.) The chapter begins with a description of a psychotherapeutic paradigm for working with individuals with HIV-related cognitive impairment. This model distinguishes between mild and more severe impairment, providing the clinician with a guide for treating a condition that can be transient, static, or progressive.

The chapter continues with a discussion of specific treatment issues and approaches for conditions that may require a psychopharmacological consultation: psychosis, mood disorders, agitation, anxiety, and substance abuse. It includes a discussion of how to coordinate treatment with psychiatrists and general principles for the use of psychoactive medications.

The Psychotherapeutic Approach

Summary

- There are two psychotherapeutic models for managing HIV-related cognitive impairment: "Adaptation and Compensation," which is used with mild cognitive impairment, and "Environmental Engineering," which is used with moderate to severe impairment. In addition, three elements of psychotherapeutic practice deserve particular attention: education, coordination of treatment, and ethical dilemmas.
- Education can foster realistic expectations about the symptoms, course, and intervention strategies of cognitive impairment and make the diagnosis less overwhelming.
- Management of cognitive impairment can be improved by a coordinated approach to care between mental health and medical providers.
- The primary ethical questions that arise in psychotherapy with clients with cognitive impairment involve safety and the therapist's dilemma over whether or not to intervene to protect the

client or a third party. Providers and caregivers may also have to decide when it is appropriate for them to substitute their own judgment for that of the client in terms of activities like driving and living independently.

Since HIV-related cognitive impairment may be stable or progressing, or episodic and transient, clients with HIV disease are best served by ongoing assessment and a flexible psychotherapeutic approach. This principle of adapting therapeutic approach to level of impairment is the foundation of the interventions discussed throughout this chapter.

There are two models for managing HIV-related cognitive impairment, both of which apply to other dementing illnesses.[57,58] The first approach – "Adaptation and Compensation" – is used with mild cognitive impairment such as HIV-associated minor cognitive/motor disorder. Interventions aim at reinforcing remaining strengths while helping individuals compensate for changes in ability. The goal of this approach is to maintain independence and self-esteem by encouraging full participation in treatment and life decisions. Supportive psychotherapy with an educational and problem-solving approach is most appropriate at this stage.

The second approach – "Environmental Engineering" – best addresses HIV-associated dementia or cognitive impairment of at least moderate degree. Individuals with dementia lose the ability to deal with the changing demands of the world and require structure to decrease fear and confusion and to ensure safety. With the progression of dementia, the therapist's role becomes more active and may even involve decision-making in the client's life. Psychotherapy at this stage involves educating caregivers, such as friends and family members, regarding management strategies and identifying community resources to create the necessary environmental structure. As cognitive impairment progresses, interventions may include individual, couples, and family therapy, as well as ongoing assessment, case management, and advocacy.

These are the primary considerations for providing psychotherapy to individuals with HIV-related cognitive impairment: the role of education; the importance of coordinating treatment with other caregivers; and the specific ethical issues involving safety and the practitioner's duty to protect. These considerations form a framework for treatment and preface the main discussion of management in this chapter. Following this preface, the chapter outlines specific interventions for mild and severe cognitive impairment.

Education

Education regarding HIV-related cognitive disorders is an important psychotherapeutic intervention that can foster realistic expectations and make the diagnosis of HIV-related minor cognitive/motor disorder, and indeed any cognitive impairment, less overwhelming. Cognitive impairment, commonly lumped under the heading of "dementia," is one of the most frightening conditions associated with HIV disease, and it may also be one of the issues clients are least likely to feel comfortable raising during therapy.[59] For clients who have observed the effects of dementia, fears revolve around the loss of control and autonomy. For clients with less experience with dementia, the term may conjure up images of violence and psychosis.

Impairment may be demystified by explaining the physical, emotional, and cognitive changes that may occur and the extent to which they can be ameliorated. Providers should clarify that these changes are organic and not within the conscious control of the client. For example, some people may interpret a client's distractibility as resulting from anxiety, or perceive memory problems as arising from disinterest or preoccupation. Similarly, in later stages of impairment, apathy may be misconstrued as depression, and cognitive inflexibility as stubbornness. Providers should emphasize that these symptoms arise from damage to the brain and not from environmental or personality factors, although these factors may exacerbate organic symptoms.

Providers should also talk about the course of impairment, although this is difficult because there is so much uncertainty about the progression of HIV infection in the brain. At present, there is no way to know if an individual with HIV-associated minor cognitive/motor disorder will subsequently develop dementia, and if so, within what time period. Providers can educate clients about what is known and possible intervention strategies for dealing with cognitive impairment.

There is a caveat to psychotherapists regarding education. Many clients want education and want to be active participants in their treatment. Others do not, preferring that their medical providers manage their disease without significant client input. Although this reaction may be due to depression or anxiety, it may also be a personality style. Psychotherapists should be aware that clients may not want factual information, at least for a period of time. However, these clients may agree to the education of their partners or family members.

Coordination of Treatment

The treatment and management of cognitive impairment will be improved by coordinating care between mental health and medical providers. It is useful to lay the foundation for such coordination early in the therapeutic relationship. Routinely obtaining releases from clients with HIV disease will facilitate a two-way exchange of information later in the course of illness.

When questions of cognitive or behavioral change arise, psychotherapists should strongly encourage clients to contact their physicians in order to rule out or treat reversible causes of impairment. Therapists can facilitate this diagnostic process by answering clients' questions about various possible disorders or about evaluation procedures. They can also reduce resistance by responding to clients' fears about the diagnostic process and the loss of functional ability that may follow cognitive changes.

If an acute psychiatric disorder develops, the nonmedical psychotherapist will need to coordinate treatment not only with the primary physician but also with a psychiatrist. Psychiatrists can provide valuable consultation about neuropsychiatric disorders and conduct diagnostic work-ups. In addition, psychiatrists coordinate hospitalizations for acute episodes of psychiatric distress and manage psychiatric medications.

Ethical Issues

The primary ethical questions that arise in psychotherapy with clients with cognitive impairment involve safety and the therapist's dilemma over whether or not to intervene to protect the client or a third party. This may be particularly true in a work situation where the client is fighting to maintain independence but, due to cognitive limitations, may be behaving in a way that threatens the safety of others. The therapist must balance his or her ethical or legal obligations to intervene with the potential harm to the client, for example, through loss of confidentiality and alienation from the therapeutic process. Alexandra Beckett and Peter Kassel offer a good example of the ethical issues that arise among clients with progressing HIV-related cognitive impairment:[60]

> In psychotherapy, an HIV-infected emergency room nurse reported with much distress an incident of giving an inaccurate dose of morphine to a patient and, further, the fact that he had included some nonsensical statements in his weekly charting. When his therapist raised the question of organic impairment, the client refused to consider this, stating that his cognitive difficulties were just residual symptoms of depression, which had been successfully treated.
>
> Although feeling some urgency, the therapist was able to empathize with the client's sense of professional responsibility and fear of being found incompetent. The therapist's patience and support allowed the client to raise the possibility of transfer to a non-patient care position, a move that the therapist stressed would both protect the patient – the overriding goal – and maintain the client's work life for as long as possible.

As cognitive impairment progresses, providers and caregivers may have to decide when it is appropriate for them to substitute their own judgment for that of the client. When cognitively impaired clients insist that they can handle their own finances, drive, or maintain a household, providers face an ethical dilemma: given limited information, how does one determine the relative value of safety versus autonomy? There is no simple answer to this conflict of values. To aid in assessment, the psychotherapist's approach should be one of information gathering. This is done through frequent consultation with members of the treatment team and periodic contact with the client's family and friends.

Mild HIV-Related Cognitive Impairment

Summary

- The Adaptation and Compensation model used to respond to mild cognitive impairment helps clients adapt by using active problem-solving and compensate for waning skills by developing new ones.
- Making realistic plans may increase a sense of control and competence. Psychotherapy can be helpful in identifying wishes for the

future and making short- and long-term plans to meet these goals.

- Psychotherapy should encourage clients to be as independent as possible by capitalizing on strengths and compensating for limitations.
- Psychotherapy provides the opportunity for clients to discuss feelings like anxiety, depression, and anger in a safe atmosphere. In addition, anxiety and depression may require referral for psychiatric medication.
- Antiviral medications, like ZDV, may lead to improvement on neuropsychological measures and neurological functioning, although clear evidence that they improve daily functioning remains to be demonstrated.

Mild impairment occurs most often in the presence of HIV-associated minor cognitive/motor impairment, which may or may not progress to HIV-associated dementia. It may also arise in the early stages of PML or as a result of lymphoma. A significant percentage of people with HIV disease develop some degree of cognitive impairment as they become progressively weaker. To facilitate clarity, this discussion will use HIV-associated minor cognitive/motor impairment as the prototype of mild impairment.

Individuals with HIV-associated minor cognitive/motor impairment have some slowness in their thinking, mild memory problems, and decreased problem-solving ability in the face of complex or novel tasks. Mild impairment, however, does not interfere with the ability to live independently or to interact meaningfully with others.

The Adaptation and Compensation model is the best approach for mild cognitive impairment. While this intervention recognizes cognitive losses, therapy focuses on helping clients adapt through active problem-solving and to compensate for waning skills by developing new ones.

Antiviral treatment – which has been shown in some studies to ameliorate impairment – is usually initiated by a primary care physician when an individual is first diagnosed with HIV-associated minor cognitive/motor disorder. Antiviral drugs like ZDV may intervene in HIV brain infection by slowing viral replication.

Realistic Goals and Active Problem-Solving

Clients with mild cognitive impairment can participate fully in decision-making and should be encouraged to do so. Making realistic plans may increase a sense of control and competence. Psychotherapy can be helpful in identifying the client's wishes for the future and making short- and long-term plans to meet these goals. Four areas of planning are particularly important: legal, medical, employment, and daily living.

Planning should include decisions about legal documents, such as wills and medical directives, that need to be undertaken in a timely fashion while clients are still considered mentally competent. Among these documents are Living Wills, which detail limits on treatment in response to the end-stage of a life-threatening disease, Wills, Durable Power of Attorney for Health, and Durable Power of Attorney for Finances. While therapists should refer clients to legal resources for help in drawing up such documents, therapists can assist in decision-making by allowing clients a forum in which to discuss difficult choices – for example, choosing people to manage their financial affairs and health care decisions. With regard to medical decisions, clients should inform both their designated appointees and their primary physicians of wishes regarding medical interventions during the terminal phase of illness or treatment preferences should they develop dementia.

Psychotherapists should document these discussions and their assessment of the patient's competence in their own chart notes. A key issue is whether or not the patient is able to understand their choices and the ramifications of their decisions.[61] For wills in particular, psychotherapists may suggest conducting neuropsychological testing during this same period in order to address any future questions regarding competency, and even videotaping the execution of the will to respond to potential legal challenges.

With regard to employment, a client may decide to modify or stop work and arrange for disability coverage when fatigue, additional medical problems, and the demanding nature of a client's job become untenable. Therapists can facilitate a discussion regarding both the decision-making process leading to a change in work patterns and the sense of loss that may accompany such a decision. During this process, therapists may be confronted with the need to be more actively involved than usual. For example, they may be asked to provide documentation regarding cognitive impairment in order for the client to receive benefits. It may also be helpful for therapists to be familiar with federal and state laws requiring an employer to "reasonably accommodate" disabled employees, that is, to modify their job duties.[61]

For clients who are no longer working, it is particularly important for practitioners to encourage planning of daily living. Adding structure to the day and incorporating activities and tasks that are achievable ensures that clients maintain a sense of accomplishment and quality of life.

Compensation

Psychotherapists should encourage individuals with mild HIV-related cognitive impairment to be as independent as possible by capitalizing on strengths and compensating for limitations. Among the compensatory strategies available to clients are the following:

- Slowing down and performing one task at a time can decrease frustration and the tendency to make mistakes.
- Getting enough rest and making appointments early in the day can minimize fatigue.
- Developing familiar routines and avoiding crowded public places or peak business hours can prevent overstimulation.
- Relaxation exercises, stress reduction techniques, and massage can reduce tension or anxiety.
- Regular exercise can also reduce stress and may result in retention of coordination and motor skills.[62]
- Adaptive devices such as appointment or memory books can document important dates, information, or conversations.
- Alarmed or compartmentalized pill boxes can aid in monitoring medication.

Emotional Responses

Anxiety, depression, and anger are common reactions to the changes wrought by mild HIV-related cognitive disorder. Clients may describe themselves as sluggish, and they may experience a decreased sense of competency and an inability to organize themselves. These experiences may lead to rational fear and anxiety about their deficits and the future. Other clients may deny their faulty perceptions and inaccurate memories, and when confronted, may become angry or depressed.[63]

Psychotherapy provides the opportunity to discuss these feelings in a safe atmosphere. Support groups may allow clients to meet others who are successfully coping with impairment and may help clients anticipate future impairment-related challenges and concerns. In addition to psychotherapy, anxiety and depression may require referral for psychiatric medication.

Emotional reactions occur not only among clients but also among their partners or families. Partners or family members may deny the existence of any deficits, stating that the client has "always been this way," or they may overreact, taking control and making decisions that the client still has the capacity to make. Couples therapy may be particularly useful in dealing with role reversals in the relationship, a change that can result in clients feeling frustrated and angry, and caregivers feeling overwhelmed, resentful, and guilty.

Suicidal thoughts and intentions may occur throughout the course of HIV disease, especially at crisis points such as the onset of cognitive impairment or the loss of control of bodily functions.[64] While there is legitimate debate in the mental health field regarding the proper clinical and ethical stance regarding suicidal clients with terminal illness, it is important that therapists carefully evaluate the psychological, social, and neuropsychological determinants of despair prior to accepting a client's view that he or she has no options for improving the quality of life. If they exist, providers should aggressively address treatable cognitive and mood disorders that may result in suicidality.

In situations where clients wish to discuss suicide as an option, clinicians would be wise to take a balanced approach. Therapists need to recognize that for many HIV-infected clients, knowing that they have the option to end their lives if they determine that the circumstances are intolerable provides hope and a sense of control. Overreacting by threatening hospitalization may serve only to increase anxiety and resistance. Instead, providers should collaborate to appropriately share decision-making with clients, in this way providing them the sense of control necessary to make a frightening situation seem bearable. Nonetheless clients usually feel reassured to know that – when they are unable to make rational decisions because of conditions such as transient psychosis, drug intoxication, or delirium – medical team members, including psychotherapists, will intervene.[59]

Antiviral Treatment

Currently, although there is no cure for HIV-associated dementia, it has been common practice to begin antiviral medication when an individual is diagnosed with HIV-associated minor/cognitive motor impairment or dementia. These medications have been used in varying doses with varying results in an effort to improve cognitive performance and slow the progression to dementia.

Studies of ZDV have generally supported its clinical use for this purpose. One small but well-designed investigation found that after taking ZDV (200 or 400 milligrams five times daily) for 16 weeks, a group of 40 subjects significantly improved their performance on a battery of neuropsychological tests when compared to a group of similar patients taking placebo. Furthermore, the improvement was sustained for a 32-week period.[65] An additional study suggests that ZDV may have a preventive effect with regard to HIV-associated cognitive impairment if it is started prior to a diagnosis of AIDS.[66] While the optimal dose of ZDV in the treatment or prevention of cognitive impairment has not been clearly determined, there appears to be greater benefit using doses higher than the standard of 600 milligrams per day, and physicians often prescribe doses of 1,000 milligrams or more per day.

Although a number of studies have reported ZDV-related improvement on neuropsychological measures and neurological functioning, clear evidence that ZDV improves daily functioning remains to be demonstrated.[67] Even accepting that early, high-dose ZDV may protect against HIV-associated dementia, it is unclear if this effect is sustainable. Two other antivirals, didanosine (ddI) and dideoxycytidine (ddC) are being used alone or in conjunction with ZDV to extend or increase its effectiveness, but there is little information to date about therapeutic response. In addition, resistance to all three medications may develop within six to twelve months.[68]

HIV-Related Dementing Conditions

Summary

- In the face of moderate to severe dementing conditions, therapy changes. The emphasis of therapy shifts from processing feelings to negotiating the practical issues of day-to-day living. The frame of the psychotherapeutic session may change in response to the client's physical limitations. The goals of therapy shift away from adaptation and more towards defining the client's increasing needs for assistance, potentially taking on a decision-making role in the client's life.

- As dementia progresses, the Environment Engineering model is the central tool for management. It is crucial to structure the client's environment in five areas: orientation, communication, memory, movement, incontinence.
- Structuring the client's environment may also prevent hazardous behavior, particularly in the following arenas: independent living, home safety, wandering, and driving.
- Emotional and personality changes – including volatility, denial, and catastrophic reactions. Management includes four crucial steps: accurate diagnosis; education of clients and caregivers to clarify that behavior is organic and not volitional; structuring the environment to eliminate confusion; and avoiding confrontation.

Dementia is a brain disorder that is significant enough to interfere with occupational or daily social functioning. While there are several causes of dementia in individuals with HIV disease, the most frequent is HIV-associated dementia. Since HIV-associated dementia is a useful prototype for all HIV-related dementing conditions, it is the focus of the discussion in this section.

HIV-associated dementia leads to memory loss, impaired manipulation and retrieval of information, and slowed thinking. Behavioral abnormalities include apathy, depression, and less frequently, manic or hypomanic symptoms. Motor impairment may begin with changes in handwriting but is most notable for leg weakness, slowed movements, balance problems, and general clumsiness. With moderate cognitive impairment, individuals are no longer able to work and may need some assistance, but can still take an active part in daily care and continue to interact with friends and family. As dementia progresses, individuals may no longer be able to live independently, and they may no longer be able to make reasonable decisions.

In response, management shifts from the Adaptation and Compensation model applied to mild cognitive impairment to the Environmental Engineering model. This model emphasizes matching the amount of structure provided with the degree of impairment present. The involvement of caregivers and health providers, and the need for community resources, increases as functional abilities decrease.

Psychotherapy

In the face of moderate cognitive impairment, psychotherapy can no longer be reflective or psychodynamic. The therapist needs to take a pragmatic and direct approach, be more generous with suggestions, and at times even give advice. The emphasis of therapy shifts from processing feelings to negotiating the practical issues of day-to-day living. A session may consist of checking in on basic competencies like the ability to plan for meals or arrange transportation, or of discussing visits with doctors and current health status.

The frame of the psychotherapeutic session may also change in response to the client's limitations. For example, the psychotherapist may suggest including the client's partner or caregiver periodically, particularly to discuss logistical problems that may arise. Clients may come less frequently as doctor's appointments, fatigue, and forgetfulness increase. At this point, psychotherapist and client might consider meeting less often or talking by telephone. While some psychotherapists are comfortable meeting at a client's residence, providers considering such alternatives must pay special attention to therapeutic boundaries.

At the level of moderate impairment, therapy shifts further away from adaptation and more towards defining the client's increasing needs for assistance, an evolution that brings about changes in the client's interpersonal relationships. To aid the client in this pursuit, the therapist should consider addressing the following questions. What kind and how much help does the client need? Can the client expect support from others? From whom specifically? What help can the therapist give, and what other resources are available in the community to meet the client's needs? Although processing emotions is not useful for clients at this level of impairment, discussing these questions and asking clients how it feels to have others take more responsibility for them can be supportive. In the course of this discussion, providers should be sensitive to clients' reactions to their increasing inability to care for themselves and, consequently, their need to rely on others.

As impairment worsens, therapy may serve to maintain a sense of continuity and support for the client and, increasingly, for caregivers. Therapists may take on the role of consultant to family and friends and facilitator between caregivers and health providers. They may be particularly helpful in facilitating a home care plan that incorporates Environmental Engineering interventions and may even become actively involved in decision-making, for example, when issues of safety arise.

The next section addresses specific treatments and management problems for clients with dementia and practical interventions that create structure and safety.[26] This section is divided into three main areas: physical and cognitive changes, safety concerns, and emotional and personality changes. Many of the problems described below, such as incontinence, are outside the usual realm of psychotherapy, but it is exactly this type of issue that may preoccupy, even overwhelm both the client and his or her caregivers and that will determine the client's quality of life.

Physical and Cognitive Changes

Educating caregivers and clients about physical and cognitive changes that occur with dementia can promote better relationships, ensure safety, and reduce stress. The particularly problematic changes and their corresponding interventions are addressed under the following topics: orientation, communication, memory, movement and incontinence.

Orientation

Individuals with dementia frequently become confused and disoriented. This may be most evident at night (this syndrome of disorientation at night is called "sundowning"). Confusion may also follow a "good day/bad day phenomenon" pattern, or vary over longer periods of time. Particularly if the onset of confusion appears acute, providers need to rule out delirium as a cause. Finally, hospitalization or any change in environment may cause or worsen confusion. To decrease confusion:

- Maintain a familiar environment by avoiding unnecessary travel, moves, or redecorating.
- Maintain a routine daily schedule.
- Too much or too little stimulation can worsen confusion or cause agitation. Modulate stimulation accordingly.

- For sundowning, use a night light or soft radio. If fatigue worsens sundowning, encourage activity in the morning and an afternoon nap.
- Provide frequent orientation cues, either verbally or by displaying clocks, calendars, or a written daily schedule.
- Prepare clients for change by walking them through a task as it occurs.
- Avoid confronting an individual's reasoning or proposed course of action. Instead redirect or distract clients from troublesome or inappropriate behavior.

Communication

Prior to late-stage dementia, verbal expression may be impaired only by slowed speech, mild word-finding problems, and a tendency to ramble or be circumstantial.

As dementia progresses, the ability to understand spoken language (also known as receptive language) becomes impaired, but this deficit may be masked by the overall fluency of a client's speech. In particular, clients may be unable to process lengthy sentences and this may lead to miscommunication. Late-stage impairment may include muteness. It is important to note that HIV infection can affect hearing and that visual problems can arise secondary to CMV retinitis. To respond to receptive language deficits:

- Before addressing the client, limit background noise, and then get the individual's attention by calling out his or her name.
- Slow down speech, and speak in simple sentences.
- Ask the client to repeat the information back to insure that he or she correctly heard and understood it.

Memory

Since memory impairment may result in missed psychotherapy sessions, it is important for therapists to recognize HIV-associated dementia in order to distinguish between memory loss and volitional or unconscious behavior, such as resistance in psychotherapy or "acting out." It can be difficult, however, to assess memory informally. Even with moderate cognitive impairment, clients retain remote memory (memory of past life events and school- or work-based knowledge), and articulate clients, in particular, may seem capable of remembering more than they actually can. Clients may also begin to "confabulate" answers; that is, they may fill in missing gaps in memory in order to create a continuous story or block of information, merging disparate events, conversations, or thoughts.

Memory impairment may lead to frustration, and to feeling disregarded, poorly treated, or even persecuted. To respond to these feelings as well as to memory loss:

- Introduce a daily routine, which decreases the client's need to rely on memory or keep track of new information.
- Remove clutter to help the client find misplaced items.
- Use a "memory book" or large wall calendar to cue recall for events and appointments. As dementia increases and clients forget to use these tools, caregivers should write down important information and cue clients to read it. With severe cognitive impairment, clients may no longer be able to do this and may become frustrated at the request.
- As memory problems worsen, clients may not remember how to navigate their living space. To cue clients, label doors and drawers with both a word describing the contents and a drawing illustrating them.
- While assessment is crucial for determining degree of impairment, it often focuses on the failure to remember. To instill a sense of security and well-being, encourage clients to talk about areas of interest and memories they have retained over time.

Movement

Increasing weakness and balance problems may limit mobility, and this may lead to a shuffling walk and a tendency to stumble or fall. Incoordination may manifest as clumsiness, poor handwriting, and difficulty manipulating buttons or zippers. The following suggestions may facilitate activities of daily living:

- Walkers and canes may help compensate for balance problems.
- Straight-backed chairs or chairs with arms aid in sitting and rising.
- A shower bench or raised toilet seat may decrease the possibility of falls.
- Adaptive equipment such as bowls with non-skid bottoms can facilitate eating.

- Individuals with severe dementia may need verbal cues or pantomimed gestures to initiate activities such as eating.

A physical or occupational therapist can help in assessing a client's abilities and initiating adaptive devices. Sudden onset of balance problems or incoordination raises the question of an acute medical problem and should precipitate referral to a physician.

Incontinence

Bowel and bladder incontinence may occur for a variety of reasons independent of HIV-associated dementia: neuropathy of the bladder or urinary tract infection, wasting syndrome, diarrhea, or end-stage HIV disease may all cause incontinence. Medication side effects or the onset of an opportunistic illness can cause incontinence, and with attendant diarrhea there may be dehydration, electrolyte imbalance, and delirium. Sudden onset of incontinence may be due to an acute condition and requires immediate medical response.

Incontinence may occur with dementia, as individuals become more fatigued or have more difficulty walking to the bathroom. Confusion may result in difficulty finding the bathroom or in urinating in inappropriate locations. As dementia progresses, individuals may no longer be aware of the need to urinate or defecate. In response to incontinence:

- Label bathrooms with verbal and visual cues.
- Place a commode by the bed.
- Limit liquids before going to bed.
- To reduce the likelihood of accidents, create a toileting schedule or have someone escort the client to the toilet during the night.
- If incontinence is an ongoing problem, use adult diapers and consult a psychiatrist about psychopharmacological treatment

Safety Concerns

Increasing memory problems, physical decrements, confusion, and organic denial can lead to hazardous behavior. Usually this becomes apparent when a client gets lost or creates a dangerous condition such as forgetting to turn off the stove burner or dropping a lit cigarette onto the floor. Safety issues are a primary concern in the following arenas: independent living, home safety, wandering, and driving.

Ability to Live Independently

With moderate cognitive impairment, individuals are generally able to live independently with some assistance, but as dementia progresses, they may no longer be able to live alone or care for themselves. Therapists should undertake ongoing assessments of the capacities of their clients to live independently by reviewing day-to-day tasks such as the abilities to shop, prepare meals, drive, pay bills, and take medication. Therapists should listen for descriptions that suggest poor judgment, hazardous situations, or getting lost. In this process, it is also useful to gather information from friends and family. A mental status examination – compared to results from a previous exam – and neuropsychological or occupational therapy evaluations may also help in determining the capability to live independently.

There are interventions that can provide support or supervision and allow a client to remain at home even as impairment worsens. Caregivers, such as partners, roommates, or family members may be able to provide supervision and manage medications. In large cities, day treatment programs specifically designed for people with HIV disease can provide structure during the day; unfortunately, in most places, only general psychiatric day treatment programs or geriatric programs may be available. In some cities, meal delivery programs, such as Meals-on-Wheels, may bring cooked meals to disabled people with HIV disease. In other locations, senior centers or religious groups may provide assistance with meals. Finally, skilled nursing programs may be available to come into the home to provide limited medical care. (See Resources, page 83, for advice on identifying local services.)

Home Safety

Health providers should discuss safety-proofing the home with clients and caregivers as another way of compensating for cognitive impairment. To increase safety:

- Decrease the risk of falling or bumping into objects by removing slip rugs and organizing furniture to provide more open space in which to maneuver.
- Provide good lighting especially in hallways and on stair landings.
- Safety proof the tub or shower by placing non-slip surfaces on

the floor. Adjust the water heater to reduce the temperature of the hot water so confusion will not lead to scalding.

- Install metal plates to cover stove burners or plastic covers for stove dials.
- Install child-proofing hardware to limit access to drawers or cabinets that house potentially dangerous substances or utensils.

Wandering

Wandering, or aimless ambulation, occurs as a result of disorientation and memory impairment. It constitutes one of the most serious management issues faced by professional and personal care givers working with cognitively impaired clients.[23]

Wandering is particularly dangerous when it occurs prior to significant physical debilitation. Individuals with wandering behavior may walk the streets until they come to the attention of social services personnel, hospital staff, or police. Finding a residential setting that can manage these clients is very difficult. Throughout the country, there may be a few metropolitan areas with a locked ward designed specifically for clients with HIV-associated dementia. Unfortunately, in most cities, individuals who wander may be placed on locked psychiatric units, which while protecting them may also exacerbate their confusion.

In many cases, however, dementia occurs along with an overall physical decline and weakness, and wandering does not constitute a significant risk in the face of home modification and appropriate supervision. To respond to the risk of wandering:

- Clients should carry identification cards and wear identification bracelets or dog tags – printed with name, address, and telephone number. Caregivers should have a recent photograph of individuals with dementia to help police locate them if they wander.
- Place a bell on an outside door to ring and sound an alert when the door is opened.
- Create barriers to wandering. Adjust doors so they are more difficult to open. Plastic door knob covers may make handles difficult to turn. An additional lock placed at the bottom of a door may be overlooked by a client with dementia and may deter him or her from exiting.

Driving

For many people, driving is a symbol of independence and for individuals with dementia, driving can be one of the hardest activities to relinquish. Caregivers, including psychotherapists, may be reluctant to take away this symbol of autonomy or be confused about when it is necessary to intervene. Sometimes the decision is made after an episode when the client gets lost. In other cases, it is after neuropsychological testing reveals dementia.

Moderate cognitive impairment leads to reduced reaction time, poor judgment, distractibility, visual-spatial problems, and difficulty performing multiple tasks at one time. In California, physicians are legally required to report dementia to their county health department which must then forward this information to the Department of Motor Vehicles. With regard to other health care providers, the law is gray. Psychotherapists should be aware, however, that if a cognitively compromised client has a motor vehicle accident, his or her therapist may face liability if the therapist has failed to file a report. Nonetheless, this is a complex matter, requiring practitioners to balance issues of confidentiality, competency, and the duty to warn.

Psychotherapists should educate caregivers about a client's deficits, and assist the client and his or her caregivers in making a decision about driving. Sometimes individuals are aware of difficulties with driving and accept the need to stop. Due to denial or poor judgment, others may have more problems accepting the decision that they are no longer safe to drive. To respond to this issue, caregivers can take the following actions:

- Distract the individual when he or she wants to drive by engaging in a discussion about other issues.
- Avoid confrontation by offering to drive as a way of allowing the client the opportunity to rest or relax.
- With clients who are difficult to deter, hide the car keys, remove the distributor cap, or lock the steering wheel.
- To increase compliance, obtain a letter from a physician recommending that the client no longer drive.

Emotional and Personality Changes

Individuals with HIV-associated dementia undergo emotional and personality changes that are directly related to brain impairment. In addition, some cognitively impaired clients may develop serious psychiatric conditions such as a psychosis or an affective disorder. Still others may have a preexisting psychiatric disorder that reasserts itself during the course of HIV disease. Accurate diagnosis of these conditions is crucial to optimal treatment.

This section briefly describes interventions for the emotional and behavioral changes, including organic denial and catastrophic reactions, that commonly accompany HIV-associated dementia. The next section addresses major psychiatric disorders, including psychosis, anxiety, and affective disorders, which often require medication and coordinating treatment with a psychiatrist.

Ironically, as cognitive impairment progresses and interferes with daily functioning, cognitively impaired individuals often become less anxious about their symptoms of progressive dementia.[59] In conjunction with their growing inability to think abstractly, to recognize complexity, or to remember distressing events (or even worries about the future), clients with dementia become less aware of changes in themselves.

Emotions as well as thinking become simplified. As a result of cognitive deficits, there is a loss of ability to distinguish among the fine nuances of emotional states and a decreased ability to sustain emotional states. Thus, although individuals with dementia can become distressed – particularly with regard to threatened changes in living situation – they lack the depth to their emotions that is seen in cognitively intact individuals.

While people with moderate cognitive impairment tend to be apathetic, they are also overly responsive to stimulation. They can become easily distracted or agitated and they have little tolerance for frustration. Emotions can be quick and intense, manifesting as sudden mood changes or as angry outbursts that resolve quickly. This changeability in emotions can be easily misunderstood by caregivers, who tend to see this behavior as volitional and often respond in kind with frustration or annoyance. Psychotherapists need to educate caregivers about the organic bases of these emotions and behaviors as well as how to manage them and their own reactions more effectively. (See Special Issues for Providers and Caregivers Dealing with Cognitive Impairment, page 73.) This can be particularly difficult when there is more than one caregiver, for example, when there are a number of home health aides working with a client.

Organic Denial

Organic denial or "anosagnosia" (a Greek term meaning "not knowing that one does not know") is a lack of awareness of deficits that is often seen in individuals with brain dysfunction. Organic denial results in poor judgment, and clients with this condition may make strikingly unrealistic statements or decisions. In response, caregivers usually try to reason with clients; however, this may lead to angry outbursts and a more entrenched position.

Organic denial cannot be addressed directly; caregivers should avoid confrontation and try to defuse the situation by being matter-of-fact and offering assistance in problem-solving. For example, when an individual with HIV-associated dementia insists that he can cook dinner, his partner offers to help rather than arguing about the client's abilities. Together, they plan the menu and, as the client's interest in the preparation wanes, the partner takes over and completes cooking.

Organic denial can be particularly hard for caregivers because it presents such a glaring example of cognitive impairment in a loved one. It also creates a situation where caregivers are increasingly responsible for a person who can no longer make rational decisions.

Catastrophic Reactions

Unable to process information, people with severe dementia tend to become easily overwhelmed and react out of proportion to the circumstances. The resulting catastrophic reactions – irritability, agitation, or outbursts of crying or anger – occur when an individual feels confounded by stimulation or frustrated by his or her inability to do a task. Among the precipitating circumstances that may set off catastrophic anxiety are: unfamiliar surroundings; too much noise; too many people; small accidents; being contradicted; being asked too many questions; being given too many choices; being left alone; feeling lost or insecure; or feeling rushed. To prevent or interrupt these reactions:

- Monitor stimulation.
- Interact in a calm manner, and approach the individual slowly.
- Allow time for the impaired individual to adjust so he or she does not feel rushed.
- Simplify tasks and present limited choices.

- Give directions one step at a time, and repeat these directions.
- Walk the individual through a task as you do it, for example, during dressing, tell him or her what you are doing.
- Avoid physical restraint if possible; this is likely to increase agitation.
- Consider medications for reducing agitation and anxiety, especially if there has been an abrupt change in environment, for example, hospitalization.

Psychosis, Anxiety, and the Affective Disorders

Summary

- Psychosis, anxiety, organic mania, and depression are all amenable to psychopharmacological treatment. Close communication between psychotherapist and psychiatrist aid in evaluation, choice of appropriate drug treatment, and accurate monitoring of drug effects.
- To respond to psychosis and anxiety, prescribing psychopharmacological treatment, and providing a routine and structured environment, and monitoring levels of stimulation may all be useful. Psychiatric hospitalization may be necessary in some instances of psychosis. Education regarding the organic nature of these conditions can reduce fear and distress among clients and caregivers.
- Treatment of organic mania requires medication and, in severe cases, hospitalization. Since mania impairs judgment, it is crucial to provide a structured environment, with supervision focusing in particular on medication compliance, until the mania is adequately treated. Psychiatric hospitalization or some other form of structured environment may be necessary until symptoms abate.
- Organic depression is less likely to be managed through psychotherapy. There are two approaches to pharmacological treatment of organic depression in clients with HIV-related cognitive impairment: psychostimulants and conventional antidepressant medications.
- Treating substance abuse is a crucial first step to managing cognitive impairment.

The significant psychiatric or behavioral symptoms that accompany HIV-related cognitive impairment require psychopharmacological medication for optimal treatment. In many clinical settings, non-medical mental health providers will continue to work with clients with psychosis, anxiety, and affective disorders following consultation with a psychiatrist and the prescription of medication. Frequent contact with clients allow therapists the opportunity to monitor the benefits and side effects of medication treatment. Close communication between the therapist and the consulting psychiatrist, especially when the client has significant cognitive impairment, can maximize the benefit of consultation and medication treatment.

This section describes current medication treatments for the psychiatric syndromes seen in clients with HIV-related cognitive impairment. It includes an introduction to the general principles of psychopharmacologic treatment, and guidelines for managing psychosis, anxiety and agitation, organic mania, and depression.

Psychopharmacological Interventions

Psychopharmacologic agents, those medicines that act on the brain to affect thinking, emotion, and behavior, can provide valuable treatment of psychiatric and behavioral symptoms seen in clients with HIV-related cognitive impairment. In particular, these medications can manage a variety of disturbing and disabling symptoms and significantly improve quality of life. Psychotherapists who work with clients with HIV infection should develop a professional relationship with psychiatrists familiar with the manifestations of HIV disease. Close communication between psychotherapist and psychiatrist will aid in a client's evaluation, choice of appropriate drug treatment, and accurate monitoring of drug effects. (See Table 3: Guiding Principles of AIDS Psychopharmacology, page 65.)

Because psychopharmacologic agents generally treat symptoms, rather than "cure" specific diseases, it is important to clearly identify target symptoms and define how provider and client will measure the effectiveness of treatment at the outset of therapy. If ineffective, an agent can be discontinued, thus avoiding unnecessary side effects. If partially effective, dosage may be adjusted to maximize benefit.

Patients with HIV-related cognitive impairment, whatever the cause, are likely to be more sensitive than usual to the effects –

Table 3. Guiding Principles of AIDS Psychopharmacology

1. Identify target symptoms and desired endpoints.
2. Specify the length of a therapeutic trial.
3. Start with low dosage and increase slowly: "Start low; go slow."
4. Monitor side effects carefully.
5. Minimize the number of different medications.

including undesirable side effects – of psychotropic medications. For this reason it is prudent to begin treatment with lower than usual dosages and to make changes gradually. Monitoring for side effects should be done regularly and carefully. Providers should specifically question patients rather than wait for patients to spontaneously identify problems that they may not realize are associated with the drugs. For example, asking a patient, "Have you been feeling more restless than usual?" may elicit, "Yes, but I thought it was due to the stress of having AIDS." The patient may be experiencing the motor side effect called akathisia, caused by antipsychotic medications.

As with all medications, the likelihood of adverse effects greatly increases with the number of psychopharmacologic agents that are used. While it is not always possible to avoid this situation, providers should minimize the number of agents used. It is also important for providers to be aware of all other medications the client is taking prior to initiating a new psychopharmacologic intervention. Whenever possible, medicines that are not clearly effective should be evaluated for discontinuation.

Organic Psychosis

Organic psychosis may develop during the course of HIV-associated dementia, usually manifesting as organic mania, but also including auditory or visual hallucinations, paranoia, delusions, and confusion. Organic psychosis secondary to HIV disease needs to be differentiated from a delirium – a transient condition that results from an acute CNS disorder or medications – or a substance-induced psychosis.

Psychopharmacological treatment can be beneficial in controlling the symptoms of psychosis. Psychiatric hospitalization may also be necessary. The hospital milieu is by its nature unpredictable and can be over-stimulating for cognitively impaired individuals, thus adding to confusion and agitation. Management techniques mentioned above – specifically, providing a routine and structured environment, and monitoring levels of stimulation – are often helpful in dealing with psychotic symptoms. In addition, increasing one-on-one time with hospital staff may be useful. Finally, education regarding the organic nature of the psychosis can reduce fear and distress among clients and caregivers.

Psychotic symptoms are best treated with antipsychotic or neuroleptic agents. The more general symptoms of agitation and anxiety are best treated with either antipsychotic or specific anti-anxiety agents, depending upon the degree of cognitive impairment involved and the severity of the client's medical condition. (See Anxiety and Agitation, page 67, for a discussion of treatment.) Despite their potential side effects, these agents are effective in reducing agitation and psychosis without worsening cognitive impairment in people who are already significantly impaired.

There are many antipsychotic agents and controversy exists about which are most appropriate for use in HIV-infected clients, especially those with dementia or other cognitive impairment. Although all agents in the antipsychotic class may be effective in treating psychotic symptoms, moderate potency medications – perphenazine (Trilafon), molindone (Moban), and thiothixene (Navane) – have been especially well-tolerated and are recommended among these clients. High potency agents – such as haloperidol (Haldol) and fluphenazine (Prolixin) – are more likely than low potency agents to cause motor side effects called "extrapyramidal symptoms" (EPS) which may include muscle spasm of the neck, general muscle stiffness, shuffling gait, arm and hand tremor, and general restlessness. On the other hand, low potency medications – such as chlorpromazine (Thorazine) and thioridazine (Mellaril) – are more likely than high potency drugs to cause sedation, lowered blood pressure, and anticholinergic effects including blurry vision, constipation, dry mouth, urinary retention, and delirium. The moderate potency medications could cause any of the above effects, but, especially in low dosages, are a good compromise between either extreme on the potency continuum.

In light of these side effects, treatment should be cautious. For example, perphenazine may be started with 4 milligrams at bedtime and slowly increased by 4 milligrams daily to achieve symptom control, as long as side effects are not problematic. Molindone may be initiated with a 10-milligram bedtime dosage and increased in a similar fashion. Although it is not necessary to give these agents more than once daily, it may be useful to divide the total into two or three doses to minimize side effects. Patients should be monitored carefully for adverse effects, as HIV disease appears to increase sensitivity to the EPS motor effects of neuroleptics. If clinicians prescribe low potency agents, they should closely monitor clients for worsening cognitive impairment resulting from anticholinergic delirium.

Anxiety and Agitation

While the antipsychotics are the only class of medication available for the treatment of psychotic symptoms, there are alternatives if the target symptoms are agitation or anxiety without psychosis. This level of anxiety and agitation can occur as a result of a dementing condition, and the behavioral management techniques – including modulation of stimulation and non-confrontational supervision – may be facilitated by anti-anxiety medications. (See Catastrophic Reactions, page 62.)

The benzodiazepines are anti-anxiety agents that provide effective relief from the subjective feeling of anxiety, as well as ameliorating the somatic components of anxiety, that is, rapid pulse, heart palpitations, hyperventilation, tremulousness, light-headedness, and sweating. Along with this therapeutic effect, the benzodiazepines cause sedation and to some degree worsen cognitive and motor performance, and should be avoided for clients who have severe cognitive deficits, where further impairment may lead to increased anxiety and agitation. In clients with mild cognitive impairment, the benzodiazepines may be used safely, but they require careful monitoring in order to detect and prevent decreased cognitive performance and behavioral disinhibition.

Among the benzodiazepines, an agent with a moderate duration of action like lorazepam (Ativan) is preferable. Initial dosing generally begins at 0.5 to 1.0 milligrams two or three times daily, with increases by 0.5 milligrams at a time to achieve therapeutic effects. Initial relief of symptoms is typically seen within an hour of administration. Avoid longer acting drugs, such as diazepam (Valium), chlordiazepoxide (Librium), and clonazepam (Klonopin) since levels of these medications may accumulate in the blood stream leading to increased side effects. Ultra-short acting agents such as triazolam (Halcion) may lead to confusion and memory loss, especially in cognitively impaired clients.

Since the benzodiazepines can lead to physical dependence within several weeks, decreasing dosage or discontinuing treatment should be done with care. Abrupt decreases or discontinuation may lead to withdrawal symptoms, including increased anxiety, insomnia, tremulousness, confusion, and seizures, and may be life-threatening. Clients with cognitive impairment may inadvertently discontinue benzodiazepine treatment after misplacing the pills or confusing them with other medications.

Buspirone (BuSpar), an anti-anxiety agent may be effective for mild to moderate anxiety and agitation in clients with cognitive impairment. This agent is well-tolerated and does not produce sedation, physiological dependence, or worsen cognitive or motor function. Dosing begins at 5 milligrams three times daily and may increase to 20 milligrams three times daily. Therapeutic effect is usually seen within two weeks of initiating treatment, a significant difference from the relatively quick onset of action of the antipsychotics and benzodiazepines.

Organic Mania

Symptoms of HIV-related organic mania include hyperactivity, impulsivity, grandiose thinking, agitation and delusions. While these symptoms closely mimic symptoms of bipolar disorder, organic mania is frequently associated with motor abnormalities, memory problems, or other signs of cognitive impairment.

Organic mania usually occurs with advanced HIV disease, and may be the presenting syndrome with either HIV-associated minor cognitive/motor disorder or HIV-associated dementia. In the acute stage of organic mania, psychotherapy is not possible because of delusions, lack of judgment, and inability to reason. Treatment consists of medication and, in severe cases, hospitalization. With hypomania (a mild form of mania), the goal is to educate the client and significant others about the condition and the importance of ongoing medication compliance. For those clients without a history of bipolar disorder, clinicians should explore the relationship between organic mania and cognitive impairment once severe manic symptoms have abated. Upon resolution of the acute manic episode, it is helpful to discuss the individual's experience of the illness and answer any questions raised.

Since mania impairs judgment, it is crucial to provide a structured environment, with supervision focusing in particular on medication compliance, until the mania is adequately treated. The type of environment depends on the severity of symptoms, and may include a locked psychiatric unit, a partial hospitalization or day treatment program, a halfway house, or simply moving in with a friend or family member. Stabilization of symptoms is particularly important with organic mania, because co-existing cognitive impairment may exacerbate poor judgment. If unaddressed, impaired judgment often leads individuals to discontinue medications needed to prevent or suppress opportunistic conditions.

Psychopharmacologic treatment of organic mania usually requires a two-pronged approach: an antipsychotic/anti-agitation medication in conjunction with a mood stabilizing agent. (See page 65, Organic Psychosis, for a discussion of the treatment of psychosis and agitation.) A mood-stabilizing agent is necessary to treat manic symptoms of elevated or irritable mood, pressured speech, grandiosity, and hypersexuality.

Divalproex sodium (Depakote) and lithium carbonate are mood-stabilizing agents that specifically address manic mood symptoms, and while both appear to be effective in HIV-infected clients, there have been no controlled studies in this patient population. Valproate (in the form of divalproex sodium) may be preferable to lithium in HIV-infected clients, since dehydration from diarrhea or poor fluid intake can quickly raise lithium in the blood to toxic levels.

Treatment with divalproex sodium should be initiated at 250 milligrams two or three times daily and gradually increased as tolerated to achieve a serum level of 50 to 100 milligrams per liter. While the medication is generally well-tolerated, side effects may include nausea and vomiting, decreased blood platelet count, liver function abnormalities, and unsteadiness. Medical providers should monitor valproate blood level, complete blood count, and liver function.

Lithium treatment is initiated at 300 milligrams two or three times daily. Serum lithium level is monitored, with subsequent dosage adjustments made (usually in increments of 300 milligrams) to achieve a level of 0.6 to 1.0 mEq/L (milliequivalents per liter). Common side effects include nausea and vomiting, diarrhea, excessive urination, and tremor. While lithium-related thyroid and kidney impairment are less common, medical providers should monitor function in these areas with regular testing.

When the symptoms of mania have resolved, clients should continue ongoing treatment with mood-stabilizing agents to prevent relapse. At the same time, it may be possible to taper and discontinue medication used to treat psychosis and agitation that arise during the acute manic episode.

Organic Depression

Cognitive symptoms associated with depression include generalized mental slowing and impaired attention and concentration, both resulting in apparent memory problems. Psychotherapy with depressed patients with mild cognitive impairment may include supportive individual therapy, as well as couples or group therapy. For patients with more serious cognitive impairment, there is an increased likelihood that depression is organic in nature, and these psychotherapeutic interventions are less likely to be helpful.

There are two approaches to pharmacological treatment of organic depression in clients with HIV-related cognitive impairment: psychostimulants and conventional antidepressant medications. Since both approaches are effective, psychiatrists and clients choose based on an assessment of specific target symptoms and potential side effects.

Although controversial, psychostimulant medications are particularly well-tolerated by clients with advanced HIV disease and significant cognitive impairment. They are especially useful in clients who have serious medical illnesses and marked motor slowing. Methylphenidate (Ritalin) and dextroamphetamine (Dexedrine) have a rapid onset of therapeutic action, usually producing improved mood and increased activity level within 24 to 48 hours. These agents have also been shown to improve cognitive performance on neuropsychological testing in people with HIV-related deficits. Treatment is usually initiated with methylphenidate at 5 milligrams twice daily no later than 1:00 PM to avoid insomnia, and increased by 5 milligrams daily to achieve a therapeutic effect. Most patients will respond at a dosage of 20 to 40 milligrams, but some may require up to 80 milligrams daily. While the process is similar for dextroamphetamine, a more potent psychostimulant, the maximum daily dosage should not exceed 40 milligrams.

After initial therapeutic effect, some clients may develop tolerance to psychostimulants. For most clients, a modest increase in dosage is sufficient to regain therapeutic benefit. Though generally safe and well-tolerated, there are no long-term studies of psychostimulant use for depression in people with HIV-related cognitive impairment. Side effects include anxiety, agitation, insomnia, and mild elevation in blood pressure and pulse. While clients with histories of stimulant abuse should not be excluded from psychostimulant treatment, close monitoring would be prudent in this client population.

Conventional antidepressant medications have been shown effective in patients with cognitive impairment and organic depression. There are a wide variety of effective agents to choose from, but the selective serotonin re-uptake inhibitors (SSRIs) – sertraline (Zoloft), fluoxetine (Prozac), and paroxetine (Paxil) – have been particularly well-tolerated with low risk of worsening cognitive impairment. Sertraline may be preferable among these drugs, due to its shorter half-life, fewer interactions with other medications, and lack of sedating effect. Dosage of sertraline typically starts at 25 to 50 milligrams each morning and may be increased up to 200 milligrams, though most patients are successfully treated with 50 milligrams daily. Unlike the rapid onset of action of the psychostimulants, conventional antidepressants require two to three weeks to show benefit. To prevent relapse, the medication should be continued for at least six months following return of normal mood.

Other available agents include the traditional tricyclic antidepressants like nortriptyline (Pamelor) and desipramine (Norpramin), and the newer agents such as venlafaxine (Effexor) and nefazodone (Serzone). Although only nortriptyline has been well-studied in patients with organic depression, it is likely that all of these drugs are effective.

A Note on Substance Abuse

While this monograph does not detail the wide-ranging and complex approaches to substance abuse treatment, it is important to note that treating addiction is a crucial first step to managing cognitive impairment in substance abusers. Drugs and alcohol exert their effects on the already vulnerable brains of HIV-infected individuals through acute intoxication, chronic use, withdrawal, or a combination of these factors. These substances also worsen existing cognitive impairment caused by HIV disease, thus confusing the clinical picture, and making it difficult to diagnose and treat HIV-related cognitive disorders.

Many substances (such as cocaine, methamphetamine, and alcohol) can cause hallucinations, which can be mitigated by antipsychotic medications. In addition, withdrawal syndromes can markedly worsen cognitive impairment and, in the case of alcohol and benzodiazepine withdrawal, may be life-threatening.

Determining the best type of treatment for the individual substance abuser must take into account personal characteristics and preferences, and level of cognitive function. Group support modalities have traditionally been the most effective. Although uncommon, an outpatient program that provides HIV-related medical treatment and drug-related services in one setting may be most helpful.[69]

4

Special Issues for Providers and Caregivers Dealing with Cognitive Impairment

Both caregivers and mental health providers face enormous challenges when working with people with HIV-related cognitive impairment. They can experience a range of reactions arising from the decline of a client, increased responsibility for a client's care, uncertainty about the course of a client's illness, and the inability to make a client well. This chapter looks at the difficulties that providers and caregivers experience and suggests approaches for coping and dealing, in particular, with stress and countertransference.

Summary

- In response to the stress brought on in caring for a client with cognitive impairment, both providers and caregivers should learn about stress management techniques and seek peer support. In addition, respite is crucial for caregivers. Finally, personal stress reduction may consist of exercise, psychotherapy, or relaxation exercises.

- Countertransference may arise in many ways when caring for people with cognitive impairment. Input from consultants may provide the distance and perspective needed to recognize and respond to countertransference reactions.

Stress and Depression

There has been increasing research into coping among caregivers – friends, partners, and family members – who care for people with HIV disease, but little specifically focused on issues relating to HIV-related cognitive impairment.[57] Studies of caregivers of people with Alzheimer's disease, however, offer some insights into the HIV-related challenges and the resulting high incidence of depression and exhaustion in this population. Caregivers are worn down by unrelenting responsibility and an ongoing sense of loss when faced daily with the diminishing recognizability of a loved one. This stress is exacerbated by HIV-related stigma, by the fact that many caregivers are themselves HIV-infected, and by the fact that the support systems for many caregivers have been decimated by the epidemic.

Given their vulnerability, caregivers need to be educated about signs of stress and depression, for example, loss of appetite, insomnia, irritability, lack of pleasure in usual interests, social isolation, and the use of alcohol or drugs to relax or insure sleep. Time-limited and ongoing psychoeducational groups for caregivers can help teach management techniques and instill a sense of support and understanding. Respite services – either short breaks provided by friends or family or longer breaks provided by skilled nursing facilities – are crucial in reducing stress. In some cities, respite may be available through day activity programs for people with HIV-associated cognitive impairment. Finally, personal stress reduction may consist of exercise, psychotherapy, or relaxation exercises.

For mental health and health providers, in addition to the risk of depression, there is a possibility of burn-out or demoralization when working with individuals with HIV-related cognitive impairment. Psychotherapists can become emotionally overwhelmed by the complexity of their clients' problems, and feel helpless in the face of progressive deterioration. They may overidentify and become excessively involved, as evidenced by the amount of time they spend thinking about the client or by the intensity of their feelings during these periods. Conversely, they may become emotionally numb and disengaged, or hypochondriacally preoccupied with their own health.

These reactions can be addressed through the stress reduction techniques noted above. Consultation regarding difficult cases can also be helpful. Most important is recognizing that mental health providers are members of a treatment team and the responsibility for providing care needs to be shared with other members.

Countertransference

Traditionally, countertransference has been defined as the conscious or unconscious emotional reaction of a psychotherapist to a client. This reaction stems from the therapist's own psychological issues rather than from those of the client, and must be monitored closely in order to provide appropriate care. Particularly in the world of HIV disease, where day-to-day care may be necessary and ongoing, countertransference reactions may also be experienced by personal caregivers, especially when stress is high.

Psychotherapy with clients with HIV and additional brain disorders is fraught with countertransference possibilities. Consultation, peer case review, and a multidisciplinary treatment approach are the most helpful tools to use to avoid the pitfalls countertransference may generate.

Non-medical psychotherapists working with HIV-infected patients with apparent cognitive changes often experience feelings of apprehension and anxiety. These cognitive changes may be due to a neuropsychiatric disorder, a systemic illness, or the beginning of dementia,[63] but subtle changes, particularly if self-reported, may be due to depression or anxiety. A lack of clarity regarding the cause of symptoms can lead psychotherapists to fear that they are either being alarmist or apathetic.

Once there is a diagnosis of HIV-related cognitive impairment, therapists may feel intimidated by the need for ongoing contact with physicians or the necessity of treating a client on medication. They may feel uncertainty about their role, either feeling isolated and primarily responsible for treating a client with problems that go beyond the scope of psychotherapy, or conversely, unimportant in the realm of the client's medical or psychiatric providers.

Psychotherapists may feel uncomfortable switching from a more traditional therapeutic style to an increasingly direct and active approach. They may face dilemmas of confidentiality and divided loyalty as clients becomes less competent and more likely to endanger themselves or others. They may fear progression to dementia, and find themselves either hyperalert for these symptoms or in denial about behavioral changes or cognitive slippage.

Working with clients who are in emotional turmoil and who are confronted with the possibility of dementia raises issues for the psychotherapists about loss, vulnerability, and mortality. This may be especially true for therapists who are HIV-infected themselves or who have unresolved issues around loss.

As individuals with dementia become increasingly impaired, they become slower mentally and have less need or interest in talking. As the impaired individual becomes more emotionally distant, the connection between the client and the psychotherapist diminishes. In response, therapists may project onto clients with moderate impairment more ability for emotional experience than is actually possible. This is especially true with clients who have been particularly bright and verbal or with whom the therapist identifies.

In these instances, the therapist may feel drawn to do more insight-oriented work and to process the client's experience of decline. But the usual goal of psychotherapy with terminally ill people – to resolve unfinished business and come to some acceptance before death – is not possible with individuals with dementia. Psychotherapists may feel robbed of the opportunity to work through issues or to attain a sense of completion that will somehow mitigate the helplessness AIDS evokes.

Finally, countertransference may arise when treating substance-using clients. These clients can be difficult to work with because drug-seeking behavior may result in antisocial acts or treatment non-compliance. This behavior may lead to anger and blame on the part of providers, lowered expectations of clients, and even termination of the therapeutic relationship.

Conclusion: Issues for the Future

THE gaps in our knowledge are the greatest barrier to diagnosing and treating impairment brought on by HIV-related brain infection. Neurological and epidemiological research are necessary to provide further understanding and, in conjunction with expanded community resources, to improve management of HIV-related cognitive disorders.

The neuropsychiatry of AIDS is relatively new leaving much to be discovered. Understanding more about the specific mechanism of HIV-related brain infection would facilitate the design of effective preventive and therapeutic agents. Similarly, epidemiological research might clarify the natural history of HIV-related cognitive impairment. We need to gain a better understanding of who is at risk for cognitive impairment and who is most likely to develop specific complications. We need to be able to predict the course of cognitive impairment more reliably: who will stabilize at HIV-associated minor cognitive/motor impairment and who will progress to HIV-associated dementia? Answers to these questions could relieve the distressing uncertainty for both clients and providers.

The current health care system pigeon-holes disorders as either medical or psychiatric and creates facilities to deal with one or the other. This approach fails to provide appropriate care to people with the neurobehavioral symptoms associated with HIV disease. We need to institute more responsive community care for people with cognitive impairment, including residential settings that offer a comprehensive range of support for different levels of cognitive impairment, day treatment programs designed for medically and cognitively compromised adults, and respite care and support networks for providers.

While these gaps in knowledge and community resources are significant, the information in this monograph presents evidence of the effective diagnostic and management tools that providers currently have at their disposal. The treatment paradigm presented here recognizes the variability inherent in cognitive impairment and enables providers to adapt interventions to the changing clinical situation. The fundamental tenets of this paradigm – the focus on diagnosis, the importance of coordinating care with other providers, the broad utility of psychopharmacological intervention, the ability to match psychotherapeutic approach with degree of impairment and the importance of doing so, and the centrality of compensatory strategies and environmental engineering techniques – place providers in a powerful position from which to mitigate the impact of cognitive impairment and improve quality of life.

References

1. Boccellari A, Zeifert P. Management of neurobehavioral impairment in HIV-1 infection. In Zegans L, Coates TJ, eds. *Psychiatric Manifestations of HIV Disease.* Psychiatric Clinics of North America, Vol. 17(1). Philadelphia: WB Saunders, 1994: 183-204.
2. Snider WD, Simpson DM, Nielsen S, et al. Neurological complications of acquired immune deficiency syndrome: Analysis of 50 patients. *Annals of Neurology.* 1983; 14(4): 413-418.
3. Navia BA, Cho ES, Petito CK, et al. The AIDS dementia complex: II. Neuropathology. *Annals of Neurology.* 1986a; 19(6): 525-535.
4. Navia BA, Jordan BD, Price RW. The AIDS dementia complex: I. Clinical features. *Annals of Neurology.* 1986b; 19(6): 517-524.
5. Working Group of the American Academy of Neurology AIDS Task Force. Nomenclature and research case definitions for neurologic manifestations of human immunodeficiency virus-type 1 (HIV-1) infection. *Neurology.* 1991; 41(6): 778-785.
6. Brew B. HIV-1 related neurological disease. *Journal of Acquired Immune Deficiency Syndromes.* 1993; 6(Suppl. 1): S10-S15.
7. Price RW, Brew BJ. The AIDS dementia complex. *Journal of Infectious Diseases.* 1988; 158(5): 1079-1083.
8. Dreyer EB, Kaiser PR, Offermann JT, et al. HIV-1 coat protein neurotoxicity prevented by calcium channel antagonist. *Science.* 1990; 248(4953): 364-367.
9. Atkinson JH, Grant I. Natural history of neuropsychiatric manifestation of HIV disease. In Zegans L, Coates TJ, eds. *Psychiatric Manifestations of HIV Disease.* Psychiatric Clinics of North America, Vol. 17(1). Philadelphia: WB Saunders, 1994: 17-34.
10. Heaton RK, Grant I, Butters N, et al. The HNRC 500 - Neuropsychology of HIV infection at different disease stages. *Journal of the International Neuropsychological Society.* 1995; 1(3): 231-251.
11. Grant I, Heaton RK. Human immunodeficiency virus-type 1 (HIV-1) and the brain. *Journal of Consulting and Clinical Psychology.* 1990; 58(1): 22-30.
12. Maj M, Satz P, Janssen R, et al. WHO Neuropsychiatric AIDS Study, cross-sectional phase II: Neuropsychological and neurological findings. *Archives of General Psychiatry.* 1994; 51(1): 51-61.
13. Levy RM, Bredesen DE. Controversies in HIV-related central nervous system disease: Neuropsychological aspects of HIV-1 infection. In Volberding P, Jacobsen M, eds. *AIDS Clinical Review 1989.* New York: Marcel Dekker, Inc., 1989.
14. McArthur JC, Hoover DR, Bacellar H, et al. Dementia in AIDS patients: Incidence and risk factors. *Neurology.* 1993; 43(11): 2245-2252.
15. Maj M, Janssen R, Fabrizio S, et al. WHO Neuropsychiatric AIDS Study, cross-sectional phase I: Study design and psychiatric findings. *Archives of General Psychiatry.* 1994; 51(1): 39-49.

16. Bornstein RA, Nasrallah HA, Para MF, et al. Rate of CD4 decline and neuropsychological performance in HIV infection. *Archives of Neurology*. 1991; 48(7): 704-707.

17. Boccellari A, Dilley JW, Chambers DB, et al. Immune function and neuropsychological performance in HIV-1 infected homosexual men. *Journal of Acquired Immune Deficiency Syndromes*. 1993; 6(6): 592-601.

18. Boccellari A, Shore M, Stroad M. Neuropsychologic assessment in HIV-related disorders. In Cohen PT, Sande MA, Volberding PA, eds. *The AIDS Knowledge Base*. Boston: Little, Brown & Company, 1994: 5-32.

19. Boccellari AA. Neuropsychology of HIV infection: A clinician-researcher perspective. Address to the 99th Annual Convention of the American Psychological Association, San Francisco, August 1991.

20. Satz P, Morgenstern H, Miller EN, et al. Low education as a possible risk factor for cognitive abnormalities in HIV-1: Findings from the Multicenter AIDS Cohort Study (MACS). *Journal of Acquired Immune Deficiency Syndromes*. 1993; 6(5): 503-511.

21. Marder K, Stern Y, Malouf R, et al. Neurologic and neuropsychological manifestations of human immunideficiency virus infection in intravenous drug users without acquired immunodefiency syndrome: Relationship to head injury. *Archives of Neurology*. 1992; 49(11): 1169-1175.

22. Satz P. Brain reserve capacity on symptom onset after brain injury: A formulation and review of evidence for threshold theory. *Neuropsychology*. 1993; 7(3): 273-295.

23. Boccellari AA, Dilley JW. Management and residential placement problems of patients with HIV-related cognitive impairment. *Hospital and Community Psychiatry*. 1992; 43 (1): 32-37.

24. Hughes CP, Berg L, Danziger WL, et al. A new clinical scale for the staging of dementia. *British Journal of Psychiatry*. 1982; 140: 566-572.

25. Lyketsos CG, Hanson AL, Fishman M, et al. Manic syndrome early and late in the course of HIV. *American Journal of Psychiatry*. 1993; 150(2): 326-327.

26. Boccellari AA. The neurobehavioral consequences of HIV-1: A clinician's/researcher's perspective. *Paper presented at the American Psychological Association, Division 40,* San Francisco, August 1991.

27. McGuire D, So YT. Intracranial disorders. In Cohen PT, Sande MA, Volberding PA, eds. *The AIDS Knowledge Base*. Boston: Little, Brown & Company, 1994: 5.7.1-5.7.13.

28. Israelski DM, Dannemann BR, Remington JS. Toxoplasmic encephalitis in patients with AIDS. In Sande MA, Volberding PA, eds. *The Medical Management of AIDS*. Philadelphia: W.B. Saunders, 1990: 241-266.

29. Dismukes WE. Cryptococcal meningitis inpatients with AIDS. *Journal of Infectious Diseases*. 1988; 157(4): 624-628.

30. Berger JR, Kaszovitz B, Post MJ, et al. Progressive multifocal leukoencephalopathy associated with human immunodeficiency virus infection: A review of the literature with a report of sixteen cases. *Annals of Internal Medicine*. 1987; 107(1): 78-87.

31. So YT, Choucair A, Davis RL, et al. Primary central nervous system lymphoma in acquired immunodeficiency syndrome: A clinical and pathological study. *Annals of Neurology*. 1986; 20(5): 566-572.

32. Cummings JL, Benson DF. *Dementia: A Clinical Approach*. Boston: Butterworth-Heinemann, 1992.

33. Krauthammer C, Klerman GL. Secondary mania: Manic syndromes associated with antecedent physical illness or drugs. *Archives of General Psychiatry*. 1978; 35(11): 1333-1339.

34. Boccellari A, Dilley JW, Shore MD. Neuropsychiatric aspects of AIDS dementia complex: A report on a clinical series. *Neurotoxicology*. 1988; 9(3): 381-390.

35. Kieburtz K, Zettelmaier AE, Ketonen L, et al. Manic syndrome in AIDS. *American Journal of Psychiatry*. 1991; 148(8): 1068-1070.

36. Nurnberg HG, Prudic J, Fiori M. Psychopathology complicating acquired immune deficiency syndrome. *American Journal of Psychiatry*. 1984; 141(1): 95-96.

37. Perry S, Jacobsen P. Neuropsychiatric manifestations and AIDS spectrum disorders. *Hospital and Community Psychiatry*. 1986; 37(2): 135-142.

38. Harris MJ, Dilip VJ, Gleghorn A, et al. New-onset psychosis in HIV-infected patients. *Journal of Clinical Psychiatry*. 1991; 52(9): 369-376.

39. van Gorp WG, Satz P, Hinkin C, et al. Metacognition in HIV-1 seropositive asymptomatic individuals: Self-ratings versus objective neuropsychological performance. *Journal of Clinical and Experimental Neuropsychology*. 1991; 13(5): 812-819.

40. Fernandez F, Levy JK, Mansell PW. Management of delirium in terminally ill AIDS patients. *International Journal of Psychiatry in Medicine*. 1989; 19(2):165-172.

41. Egan V, Brettle RP, Goodwin GM. The Edinburgh cohort of HIV-positive drug users: Pattern of cognitive impairment in relation to progression of disease. *British Journal of Psychiatry*. 1992; 161: 522-531.

42. Handelsman L, Aronson M, Maurer G, et al. Neuropsychological and neurological manifestations of HIV-1 dementia in drug users. *Journal of Neuropsychiatry and Clinical Neurosciences*. 1992; 4(1): 21-28.

43. Karasic DH, Dilley JW. HIV-associated psychiatric disorders: Clinical syndromes. In Cohen PT, Sande MA, Volberding PA, eds. *The AIDS Knowledge Base*. Boston: Little, Brown & Company, 1994: 5-30.

44. Strub RL, Black FW. *Mental Status Examinations in Neurology*. 3rd ed. Philadelphia: FA Davis, 1993.

45. Leary M, Zeifert P. Clinical evaluation and management of HIV dementia. In Cohen PT, Sande MA, Volberding PA, eds. *The AIDS Knowledge Base*. Boston: Little, Brown & Company, 1994: 5-33.

46. Boccellari A, Davis A, Dilley JW. Preliminary findings on a screening checklist for HIV dementia. *Presentation from the V International Conference on AIDS*, Montreal, Canada, 1989.

47. Bocccellari AA, Dilley JW, Davis A, et al. The Neuropsychiatric AIDS Checklist: Its relationship to HIV status, immune functioning and performance. *Presentation from the VI International Conference on AIDS*, San Francisco, June 1990.

48. Stern Y, Marder K, Bell K, et al. Multidisciplinary baseline assessment of homosexual men with and without human immunodeficiency virus infection. *Archives of General Psychiatry*. 1991; 48(2): 131-138.

49. Wilkins JW, Robertson KR, Snyder CR, et al. Implications of self-reported cognitive and motor dysfunction in HIV-positive patients. *American Journal of Psychiatry*. 1991; 148(5): 641-643.

50. Lezak M. *Neuropsychological Assessment*, 2d ed. New York: Oxford University Press, 1983.

51. Zachary RA. *Shipley Institute of Living Scale.* Los Angeles: Western Psychological Services, 1986.

52. Reitan RM, Wolfson D. *The Halstead-Reitan Neuropsychological Test Battery: Theory and Clinical Interpretation,* 2d ed. Phoenix: Neuropsychology Press, 1993.

53. Wechsler E. *Wechsler Adult Intelligence Scale-Revised.* New York: Psychological Corp., 1981.

54. Buschke H. Selective reminding for analysis of memory and learning. *Journal of Verbal Learning and Verbal Behavior.* 1973; 12(5): 543-550.

55. Russell EW. Renorming Russell's version of the Wechsler memory scale. *Journal of Clinical and Experimental Neuropsychology.* 1988; 10(2): 235-249.

56. Weizel L, Boll TJ. *Short Category Test, Booklet Format.* Los Angeles: Western Psychological Services, 1987.

57. Boccellari A. Assessing and diagnosing AIDS dementia complex. In *AIDS Dementia Complex Training Manual.* San Francisco: Family Survival Project, 1990.

58. Mace N, Rabins P. *The 36-Hour Day.* Baltimore: John Hopkins University Press, 1981.

59. Goldblum P. Personal Communication. April 28, 1995.

60. Beckett A, Kassell P. Neuropsychiatric dysfunction: Impact on psychotherapy with HIV-infected gay men. In Cadwell SA, Burnham RA, Forstein M, eds. *Therapists on the Front Line; Psychotherapy with Gay Men in the Age of AIDS.* Washington, DC: American Psychiatry Press, 1994: 147-162.

61. Wood GJ, Marks R, Dilley JW. *AIDS Law for Mental Health Professionals.* San Francisco: UCSF AIDS Health Project, 1990: 79-86.

62. Lezak M. Living with the characterologically altered brain injured patient. *Journal of Clinical Psychiatry.* 1978; 39 (7): 592-598.

63. Abramowitz S, Cohen J. The psychodynamics of AIDS: A view from self psychology. In Cadwell SA, Burnham RA, Forstein M, eds. *Therapists on the Front Line: Psychotherapy with Gay Men in the Age of AIDS.* Washington, DC: American Psychiatry Press, 1994: 205-221.

64. Goldblum P, Moulton J. HIV disease and suicide. In Dilley JW, Pies C, Helquist M, eds. *Face to Face; A Guide to AIDS Counseling.* San Francisco: UCSF AIDS Health Project, 1989: 152-164.

65. Sidtis JJ, Gatsonis, C, Price RW, et al. Zidovudine treatment of the AIDS Dementia Complex: Results of a placebo-controlled trial. *Annals of Neurology* 1993; 33(4): 343-349.

66. Hamilton JD, Hartigan PM, Simberkoff MS, et al. A controlled trial of early versus late treatment with zidovudine in symptomatic human immunodeficiency virus infection. *New England Journal of Medicine.* 1992; 326(7): 437-444.

67. Everall IP. Neuropsychiatric aspects of HIV infection. *Journal of Neurology, Neurosurgery, and Psychiatry.* 1995; 58(4): 399-402.

68. McArthur JC, Selnes OA, Glass JD, et al. HIV dementia: Incidence and risk factors. In Price RW, Perry SW, eds. *HIV, AIDS, and the Brain.* New York: Raven Press, 1994: 251-272.

69. Batki S, Sorenson J. Systems of care for HIV-infected injection drug users. In Cohen PT, Sande MA, Volberding PA, eds. *The AIDS Knowledge Base.* Boston: Little, Brown & Company, 1994: 4-11.

Resources

Programs for Providers

AIDS Research and Education Program, Wayne State University, 2727 Second Avenue, Suite 142, Detroit, Michigan 48201, 313-962-2000.

Provides HIV-related education and training to all categories of health care practitioner through conferences, in-service trainings, and clinical courses. Includes training on neurological impairment.

New York University AIDS/SIDA Mental Hygiene Project, Department of Health Studies, School of Education, 35 West Fourth Street, Suite 1200, New York, New York 10012-1172, 212-998-5614.

Provides training, technical assistance, and support services in neuropsychiatry, substance abuse, and related issues for mental health providers and caregivers working with HIV disease.

Nursing Office for HIV and Mental Health, American Nurses Association, 600 Maryland Avenue, Southwest, Suite 100 West, Washington, DC 20024-2571, 202-651-7000.

Offers HIV-related education and training for psychiatric and mental health nurses. Also offers "Train the Trainer" services and a general education curriculum.

San Francisco General Hospital Neuropsychology Services, Department of Psychiatry, Suite 7G, Box 0852, San Francisco General Hospital, San Francisco, California 94110, 415-206-5070.

Provides training regarding diagnosis, treatment, and management of patients with HIV-related neurological impairment.

UCSF AIDS Health Project, Box 0884, San Francisco, California 94143-0884, 415-476-6430.

Provides training, consultation, and written materials on HIV-related mental health and counseling, including the response to HIV-related cognitive impairment.

Programs for Caregivers

Family Care Giver Alliance, 425 Bush Street, Suite 50, San Francisco, California 94108, 415-434-3388, 800-445-8106 (800-number for California only).

Provides support and assistance to caregivers of brain-impaired adults and resource information regarding neurological impairment.

Home Care Companions, 584 Castro Street, Box 379, San Francisco, California 94114, 415-824-3269.

Offers a monthly 15-segment course teaching home care management to partners, family members, and friends of people with HIV disease.

Direct Service Programs

Robert B. Anderson Unit, Department of Psychiatry, Massachusetts General Hospital, Fruit Street, Wang 812, Boston, Massachusetts 02114, 617-726-6772.
Provides general psychiatric and neuropsychiatric evaluations and treatment for HIV-infected clients.

St. Mary's AIDS Dementia Unit, 450 Stanyan Street, 4 South, San Francisco, California 94117, 415-750-4976.
Employing a multidisciplinary staff, provides rehabilitative services for HIV-infected people with moderate to severe dementia regarding psychosocial, medical, and physical issues.

San Francisco General Hospital Neuropsychology Services, Department of Psychiatry, Suite 7G, Box 0852, San Francisco General Hospital, San Francisco, California 94110, 415-206-5070.
Offers support groups for family members and caregivers of individuals with HIV-related dementia.

Professional Referrals

American Academy of Neurology, 2221 University Avenue South East, Suite 335, Minneapolis, Minnesota 55414, 612-623-8115, 612-623-3404 (fax).
Provides referrals to members with expertise in neurological impairment and HIV disease.

Identifying Resources for Clients

Large metropolitan areas have some established community resources for individuals with HIV disease, although services for people with additional cognitive impairment are likely to be scarce. In smaller cities or more rural areas, psychotherapists will need to be creative to find appropriate psychiatric, legal, or social service referrals for their clients. The following strategies may assist in the process of identifying and accessing resources:

- County public health department AIDS offices and county hospitals can provide information about medical, psychiatric, and community resources for clients with HIV disease.
- The American Medical Association, or state or county medical associations, may list physicians who specialize in HIV disease.
- Local gay and lesbian community organizations are usually able to provide referrals to HIV-related programs and health providers.
- Organizations that provide services for indigent people may have listings of community resources for people with HIV disease.
- Local hospices are likely to know about supervised residential programs. Visiting nurses programs can provide temporary in-home care.
- County conservatorship offices or social security offices can provide information on HIV-specific legal issues.
- County departments of social services can provide financial and benefit information for people with HIV disease.

Index

UCSF AIDS Health Project Publications

	PRICE	X	QUANTITY	=	TOTAL
AIDS and the Impact of Cognitive Impairment	$7.95	x	______	=	______
The Effects of AIDS on the Brain	$.65	x	______	=	______

Prepared for families, friends, and caregivers, this brochure examines the neurological symptoms of HIV infection and offers information on the management of people with these symptoms.

$.45 each for quantities of 25 - 249	x	______ =	______
$.40 each for quantities of 250 - 499	x	______ =	______
$.35 each for quantities of 500 or more	x	______ =	______

Face to Face: A Guide to AIDS Counseling	$16.95	x	______	=	______

In this anthology, a standard in its field, 50 pioneers in HIV-related counseling survey the mental health aspects of AIDS and offer practical advice in response to the epidemic's psychosocial dilemmas.

Risk and Recovery: AIDS, HIV and Alcohol	$16.95	x	______	=	______

A handbook about the connections between alcohol use and HIV disease that offers a mixture of practical knowledge and historical and cultural perspectives to help providers approach counseling.

AIDS Law for Mental Health Professionals	$19.95	x	______	=	______

This book explores the legal and ethical issues confronting therapists when they treat people with concerns about HIV disease. Focuses on California law, but relevant to practitioners everywhere.

FOCUS: A Guide to AIDS Research and Counseling

Since 1985, this monthly newsletter has reviewed the counseling aspects of AIDS comprising an indispensable reference for the counselors, health providers, and scholars who read it.

Individual Subscription	$36.00	x	______	=	______
Individual foreign	$48.00	x	______	=	______
Institutional Subscription	$90.00	x	______	=	______
Institutional foreign	$110.00	x	______	=	______
Shipping *(no shipping for* ***FOCUS****)*	*$4.00 first item*	x	______	=	______
	$1.00 each additional item	x	______	=	______
Sales tax *(no tax for* ***FOCUS****)*	*CA residents only add 8.5%*	x	______	=	______
Payment	*Total*			=	______

❑ ***Check enclosed*** *(Please make check payable to UCSF AIDS Health Project)*

❑ ***VISA*** ❑ ***MasterCard*** ACCOUNT NUMBER ______________________

EXPIRATION DATE ______________ SIGNATURE ______________________

❑ ***Bill me*** *(net 30 days)* PURCHASE ORDER NUMBER ______________________

SIGNATURE ______________________

NAME ______________ DAY PHONE ______________

TITLE ______________ ORGANIZATION ______________

ADDRESS ______________ CITY/STATE/ZIP ______________

Mail orders: *UCSF AIDS Health Project, Box 0884, San Francisco, CA 94143-0884*

Fax orders: (415) 476-7996. ***For further information call:*** (415) 476-6430. [MS1]